How to Overcome Eating Disorders

How to Overcome Eating Disorders

Breaking Free for a Better Life

Louise V Taylor

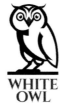

WHITE
OWL

First published in Great Britain in 2017 by
Pen & Sword White Owl
an imprint of
Pen & Sword Books Ltd
47 Church Street
Barnsley
South Yorkshire
S70 2AS

ISBN 978 1 47389 504 1

Typeset in Meta by
Mac Style Ltd, Bridlington, East Yorkshire
Printed and bound in the UK by CPI Group (UK) Ltd,
Croydon, CR0 4YY

Pen & Sword Books Ltd incorporates the imprints of Pen & Sword Archaeology, Atlas, Aviation, Battleground, Discovery, Family History, History, Maritime, Military, Naval, Politics, Railways, Select, Transport, True Crime, Fiction, Frontline Books, Leo Cooper, Praetorian Press, Seaforth Publishing and Wharncliffe.

For a complete list of Pen & Sword titles please contact
PEN & SWORD BOOKS LIMITED
47 Church Street, Barnsley, South Yorkshire, S70 2AS, England
E-mail: enquiries@pen-and-sword.co.uk
Website: www.pen-and-sword.co.uk

Contents

Chapter 1	Introduction	1
Chapter 2	Exploring Different Types of Eating Disorders	8
Chapter 3	Understanding Eating Disorders	14
Chapter 4	Health Risks Associated with Eating Disorders	22
Chapter 5	Our Cultural Emphasis on Body Image	27
Chapter 6	Biological Causes	33
Chapter 7	Environmental Factors that Increase an Individual's Risk of Developing Eating Disorders	40
Chapter 8	Conventional Treatments	52
Chapter 9	New and Developmental Treatments	64
Chapter 10	Complementary Therapies	69
Chapter 11	Nutrition and Health	75
Chapter 12	Adjusting to Change	87
Chapter 13	Breaking Free from the Lure of Pro-ana Communities	91
Chapter 14	Recovery Strategies	94
Chapter 15	The Therapeutic Effects of Writing	105
Chapter 16	How Should Parents and Families Respond?	108
Chapter 17	Jennai Cox	110
Chapter 18	Sarah's Battle with Anorexia Nervosa	113
Chapter 19	My Struggle with Bulimia Nervosa	121
Chapter 20	Hope for a Brighter Future	131
Acknowledgements		132
A Selection of Books That You Might Find Helpful		133
Index		134

Chapter 1

Introduction

E ating disorders are a growing problem in the western world, where there's a culture of individualism and considerable emphasis on the importance of appearance. In developing countries, where food shortages and famine are more common, eating disorders are very rare. So is it our culture that's to blame? Where people starve in a land of plenty?

That's certainly part of the story, but eating disorders actually go much deeper than concerns about body image. They're a sign of inner turmoil, emotional struggles, and it's often said that by controlling their bodies, sufferers feel more in control of their lives. The illness may be an expression of repressed inner pain that has been bottling up for years.

So why is the problem growing and what can we do about it? This book sets out to explore different theories, scientific studies and real life experiences relating to eating disorders. The aim is to offer information, comfort and support to those affected by eating disorders and to assist sufferers on the road to recovery.

While eating disorders have been around for decades, in recent years they have become increasingly common, seeing a 15 per cent rise between the years 2000 and 2009. They affect people of all ages, and from all backgrounds.

A survey published in the *International Journal of Eating Disorders* in 2012, found symptoms of eating disorders in 13 per cent of women over the age of 50. So although the disorders are more common among young people, they're certainly not the only group affected. Indeed, young children are increasingly developing eating disorders as they feel the pressure to meet a Western ideal of beauty. There's also been a surge in the number of men succumbing to eating disorders. The shame of the disease keeps it hidden from society and can make getting accurate data difficult. It's a secretive illness and often, sufferers are afraid of being judged, so they're reluctant to reveal the truth about their condition.

In 2015, the eating disorder charity, Beat, commissioned research by Pricewaterhouse Cooper, which concluded that 725,000 people in the UK are affected by eating disorders. In 2007, NHS researchers stated that up to 6.4 per cent of adults showed signs of having an eating disorder, and that up to 25 per cent of these people were male. Eating disorder related hospital admissions rose 8 per cent in 2014 compared to the previous year. It's clearly a big problem.

The causes of the eating disorder epidemic are many and varied, but underlying issues typically include severe self-esteem issues, depression, loneliness, and a longing to fit in and be accepted by our peers.

Our modern society can feel like a cold and uncaring place. People can be unduly critical, judgemental and unkind, offering ridicule rather than help, belittlement rather than direction. Being on the receiving end of endless criticism can erode your sense of self-worth; it's not always easy to walk away.

Furthermore, having a vocation is important, so if you can't find work, fulfilling hobbies, or another meaningful occupation, the long empty days, possibly accompanied by countless rejection letters from employers, can erode your self-esteem. Some individuals just don't feel valued.

It's also common for people to feel stressed or overwhelmed by the pace of modern life. Everyone's so busy. You might get carried along, or left behind. Either way, some individuals feel that their life is out of control. They might have emotional problems and feel there is no-one they can turn to. Controlling their body gives them some semblance of control over their lives, and might provide an emotional lift – a sense of achievement.

It's common for young people to experience a longing to be socially accepted if they've been bullied, abused, or treated like an outcast for years. Body image is often the first line of defence if we feel under attack, are called nasty names and told we need to try harder to fit in.

A background of bullying, abuse or neglect is common among people with eating disorders. Everyone needs to feel valued, feel that they are worth something, accepted by society and appreciated occasionally. Sufferers might feel torn apart by unrequited love, crushed by bullies, or just feel empty, lonely, unfulfilled and unable to change their circumstances. The range of underlying emotions and difficulties can be diverse and wide-ranging.

In an ideal world, our happiness should not depend on the love or approval of other people. But the world is not ideal and, in reality, most people would agree that they need to feel valued by someone else. So when this need is unmet, some individuals are prepared to go to extreme lengths in pursuit of peer approval, self-worth, society's acceptance, or good old-fashioned love. In an environment where body image is valued so highly, this often plays out as an obsession with appearance. In reality, it's often in pursuit of a higher goal: happiness.

Anorexia and bulimia are often triggered by attempts at slimming, to meet society's ideals. Individuals are then driven to continue by that glowing sense of achievement, pride and social acknowledgement that you get from success. Society loves people who take pride in their appearance and puts them on pedestals. Slimmers of the Year are looked up to as inspirational role models. Books on slimming are best sellers all year round. There are dozens of fad diets. Magazines are constantly promoting weight-loss. It's a billion dollar industry worldwide.

It's true that if you're overweight then slimming can be good for your health, but only if it results in healthy lifestyle changes, permanently. Yoyo diets can actually cause an increase in weight and they're demoralising. Yoyo dieting is a destructive pattern that many slimmers get into, and it can lead to bulimia nervosa, an overwhelming compulsion to binge and purge, disposing of the food you've eaten.

Once slimming becomes an obsession, it takes on a whole new life of its own. It can be emotionally rewarding on many levels – not just the sense of achievement, but by reducing your internal conflicts about being 'good enough', lovable and attractive. Fast and dramatic weight loss can numb inner pain and an obsessive focus on food can make the causes of angst and unhappiness seem less important. When you're starving, you become anaesthetised to emotional pain. The strength of feelings fades quickly, making you less vulnerable to being hurt. Your sex drive fades away and your need for companionship lessens, so you start to feel better if your social needs are unmet. It doesn't matter any more. You feel more independent.

The more weight is lost, the more emotionally detached you become. It makes you feel less exposed and you can't be so hurt by what life throws at you. For someone who's been struggling with painful emotions, this can be a relief. You feel stronger and more able to cope. You just don't feel so bad. Some experts say that starvation actually creates a sense of euphoria, as brain chemicals combine to create sensations similar to those of being on morphine.

Physiologically, extreme weight loss can result in hormonal crashes that cause a cease in menstruation and numb your sex drive, radically reducing the loneliness and pain you feel from being so alone. Individuals become so obsessed with food and their weight, that they have little time for anything else. They withdraw from their interests, go into solitude and often lose interest in relationships. But eating disorders have health consequences too.

A psychological disorder with dangerous physical implications

While some people may hold the view that eating disorders are just expressions of vanity, it actually goes much deeper than that. An eating disorder is fundamentally a psychological disorder and this is what makes it so difficult to treat. Some people do reach weights which they can see are unattractive, yet they continue to restrict their food, because they feel better that way. Understanding the long-term consequences of eating disorders can help sufferers find the strength to break free.

Very low body weight causes a drop in female hormones and a cease in menstruation. This puts some women with eating disorders at a high risk of osteoporosis in later life. Disordered eating and nutrition can also adversely affect fertility and cause reproductive problems.

One study showed that eating disorders could cause serious eye damage, possibly leading to an increased risk of blindness, or compromised vision. Sufferers may experience problems with dehydration and very poor skin condition. Dehydration can lead to kidney failure, which can be fatal. Fungal infections are more likely to occur and these can be extremely upsetting and difficult to treat.

Bingeing can cause rupture of the stomach, which can be fatal. Constipation is a common problem and there's a risk of irritable bowel syndrome whereby abdominal pain continually recurs, accompanied by constipation and/or diarrhoea. Abdominal distention and bloating supports the sufferer's impression that they're fat. Vomiting may make tiny red spots appear around the eyes, caused by burst blood vessels. When stomach acid hits your teeth, it causes slow erosion of your tooth enamel. Serious tooth decay is not pretty and costs a fortune to fix.

Skin becomes dull, dry and unhealthy in appearance. Salivary glands swell up making the face puffy, which although painless, makes the sufferer think that they have a plump face. Fasting and prolonged dieting causes sensitivity to cold and hypothermia. Low blood pressure leads to dizziness, weakness, nausea, and blurred vision.

Many people with eating disorders are at risk of a lifetime of ill health, with permanent organ damage, because in the absence of food, the body will start using its own tissues for energy. The result is a risk of life-threatening health problems, including heart weakness, kidney failure and liver damage.

Then, on top of all that, the precise balance of minerals, vital for the body to function properly, becomes altered. Malnutrition in people with eating disorders causes muddled thinking, difficulty problem solving and it makes it more difficult to make the right choices for a brighter future.

The abuse of laxatives causes metabolic disturbances, stomach cramps, water retention on stopping use and damage to the muscles that line the bowels. Chronic diarrhoea causes malabsorption, so very little of the nutrition stays in the body, making the sufferer more susceptible to disease. Malnutrition also causes exhaustion and the severest cases can go into stupor, coma and, finally, death. Eating disorders result in more deaths than any other psychiatric disorder. Beat says that around 20 per cent of anorexics die from their illness.

Laxative abuse can lead to 'lazy bowel', a potentially permanent condition, which, for those affected, presents a daily battle. The symptoms are severe constipation, abdominal pain and bloating. Toxins build up in the intestines, increasing the risk of bowel cancer and other diseases. So the sooner laxative use is stopped and healthy eating begun, the greater the chance of avoiding this condition.

Making you better again

For sufferers of eating disorders, losing some of the best years of your life to mental illness is just so sad. When you should be out in the world making your dreams come true, you're worrying about food, weight, and living in an insular world of depression. You need to learn to love yourself, overcome the obsession with weight, look outwards and break free from this downward spiral. I hope this book will help you find the strength and willpower to do that.

We're going to look at the science, the facts, backgrounds, circumstances and influences that might lead to an eating disorder. But more importantly, we'll look at how to help you, or your loved one, break free.

We'll look at treatments and the latest science. There's a section on understanding nutrition, so that you can give yourself permission to eat and not worry about the impact on your weight or appearance. Understanding nutrition can be really helpful in aiding your recovery.

We'll break down the experiences of anorexics, bulimics and those who feel out of control, so you don't feel so alone and we'll identify areas of muddled thinking and aim to address the root causes of your condition. There are many different scientific, nutritional and psychological theories around the causes of eating disorders and we'll discuss some of these and the treatments available.

You may want to seek talking therapies, or other therapies to help you, or your loved one, recover. We'll look at different therapies. Indeed, a supportive environment can be key to recovery.

If you're part of the pro-ana culture we'll look at that too, identify and discuss unhealthy perspectives and discuss how to break away from this so that you can find healthy alternative interests and start to feel better. Importantly, we'll look at how you can start engaging with society again in a positive way. You'll need other things to focus on when you start to let go of your obsession with weight, so we'll find positive alternatives to help you build confidence and good health, at your own pace.

When I talk about 'you', I mean the sufferer. If you're actually a carer, parent, partner, or a concerned citizen, that's fine too. This book is for anyone who's interested in learning more about eating disorders. But for me, it's just helpful to sometimes address the sufferer directly, as 'you'.

My background

In the mid-1990s, at the age of 20, I was recovering from anorexia and bulimia, contemplating the values of a culture in which I'd developed an eating disorder that might have killed me. Long periods of anorexia and bulimia had engulfed my life for almost five painful years. And while my peers found partners, cosied up in romantic twosomes, moved away to study, or worked in well-paid jobs they enjoyed, I'd been on a killer diet, couldn't find employment and felt exploited on a training scheme, which made things seem even worse. I'd been throwing up down the loo regularly. I'd been terrified of food, worried sick about my weight and convinced no-one would ever love me. I'd been a total mess.

For decades, I'd felt that the culture I lived in was cold, selfish and exploitative. I grew up in the 1980s, where yuppies, big hair, shoulder pads and excesses were the name of the game, but my life reflected none of that. It was an era of great hope and aspiration for many, but I grew up bullied, penniless and desperately unhappy. Most of my dreams and aspirations had been crushed before I even left school; the rest were crushed within months of leaving. Eating disorders were in the news – Princess Diana had one, and so did everyone else, it seemed. The *Daily Mail* was filled with information on the topic. The kids at school made throwing up seem normal.

My first boyfriend, who dumped me on Christmas Eve, a few weeks after my sixteenth birthday, told me I was fat – repeatedly. I was size 14 in UK sizes. Not huge. But I thought that losing some weight might solve some of my problems, making me more acceptable to my peers and more attractive to eligible young men. For years I'd longed for a boyfriend, so the fact that the only lad who'd ever paid me any attention said I was fat, was quite a big deal.

I started on a strict diet and felt good when I lost some weight. People were nice to me. Complimentary. I became addicted to it. This was, after all, the only thing in my life that was going well. So I focused on my weight and became obsessed with it.

After leaving school, I'd tried to get a job and make something of myself, but the 1990 recession had set in that April and by June, everyone was making redundancies, not hiring. I couldn't find work. I was prepared to do anything and only expected to get a job in a shop, but I couldn't even manage that. I was exhausted, broken and desperate to be loved. I was lonely. I felt lost, unwanted, undervalued. Over many months, strict dieting turned to anorexia. Ten months later, I binged. I was starving.

I panicked. I felt like I'd eaten a horse. Everything was ruined! That was the start of my bulimia. I recalled the girls at middle school, many years earlier, who practically issued instructions on how to be sick for weight control. I was only going to do it once. I mean, you wouldn't do it more than once would you? It's revolting!

But years of eating disorder obsession ensued. My body started to give up when I came close to six stone. I experienced temporary blindness. Towards the end, I realised it was causing more problems than it solved. Giving up was one of the hardest things I've ever done. But I went on to study psychology at Brunel University and I later went on to study nutrition.

Fast forward to the present day and the numbers of people with eating disorders are spiralling. So are rates of depression. We have unprecedented levels of people with mental health needs and a health service unable to cope with demand. There's a stigma around mental health and I wonder whether, in twenty years, we've actually made any progress at all.

So what's the root cause? What can be done about it? How can you rise above peer pressure? And ignore companies spending millions on exploiting your insecurities to shift products? It's become crazier in recent years, because while back in the 1980s, cosmetic surgery was the domain of the rich and famous (Cher had it routinely, not the girl next door), now it's normal among everyday folk – all because of that pressure to be perfect.

This book will help you to understand what drives people to develop an eating disorder, to understand the nature of the different conditions and I'll be suggesting approaches for recovery. I'd like to think readers will experience hope for a better future and I'll try to provide strength and encouragement to help those who feel trapped in the grip of an eating disorder, to break free and conquer the disease.

We'll be looking at anorexia, bulimia, combinations of both, and compulsive overeating. Case studies are included to help you know that you are not alone, to bring different perspectives to the table and to help readers in a caring role to empathise.

Chapter 2

Exploring Different Types of Eating Disorders

Eating disorders can develop when eating behaviour becomes obsessive, detrimental to health, or perceived as a problem. It's more extreme than just being fussy. Eating disorders are often characterised by erratic, compulsive, dangerous, or restrictive eating behaviours and they may pose a serious health risk.

Eating disorders come in many different guises, from starvation to compulsive overeating. Many people who have eating disorders don't fit neatly into one category. It's not uncommon for anorexia to lead to bulimia, for individuals to switch between the two, or for other variations of disordered eating to develop. Here we look at some of the specific disorders recognised by the medical profession and how they correspond to an individual's eating behaviour.

Anorexia

Anorexia, or anorexia nervosa, typically describes a psychological condition whereby someone is deliberately restricting their food intake, to the point of starvation, in a desperate attempt to lose weight, or maintain a very low body weight. Some definitions say anorexia is diagnosed when someone weighs less than 85 per cent of their 'expected body weight'. Others say that 25 per cent below a normal height/weight ratio qualifies as anorexia.

In anorexia nervosa, the individual will often refuse to eat, or consume very little. They might make themselves sick or take laxatives after a meal, to try to control their weight. Anorexia nervosa is the correct medical term for this psychological disorder, which distinguishes it from another form of anorexia that simply manifests as a loss of appetite for food. Loss of appetite might be caused by medication, depression, bowel problems, or a variety of other conditions, so it's not necessarily driven by the same factors as anorexia nervosa.

Some experts say that anorexics may binge and purge, like bulimics do. The key difference between the two then, is that an anorexic is underweight and a bulimic is a 'normal' weight.

The physical symptoms of anorexia nervosa might include:

- Dramatic weight loss
- Distorted perceptions of their weight and body size
- Excessive exercising
- Vomiting and/or laxative abuse
- Isolation and loss of a social life
- Emotional, irritable behaviour
- Sleep disturbances, insomnia and fatigue
- Cease in menstruation
- Extreme perfectionism
- Low blood pressure, poor circulation and feeling cold
- Growth of fine downy hairs all over the body

Some anorexics become hyperactive and restless. Others are too tired to do anything and physically, they just want to sleep. Life might demand more of them and then everything's hard work. The symptoms of starvation can make everything worse. Constipation makes them feel full and fat, abdominal cramps cause intense pain and low blood pressure and low blood sugar can cause dizzy spells. Starvation can also cause swelling in parts of the body, which might perpetuate a perception that the individual is 'fat'. The growth of fine hairs, called downy hair, on the body may occur in the severest cases, accompanied by a loss of head hair. Poor circulation causes sensitivity to the cold. The condition of the skin suffers, becoming dry and rough.

Addressing any underlying emotional traumas and slowly easing the anorexic into a more healthy pattern of eating will help to eliminate distorted impressions.

Anorexia affects people of all ages, from the very young to the very old – although often for quite different reasons. It's more common among adolescent females, although an increasing number of people from all age groups, including males, are succumbing to the disease.

Sufferers are often highly motivated, determined and ambitious individuals who believe personal achievement is important, although the disease occurs in all parts of society.

Anorexics often give the impression of being highly efficient, confident, and well organised, but deep down, they're often insecure and afraid that no matter how hard they try, they'll never be good enough. This plays out in their characteristic of perfectionism. They're addicted to achievement; success is never enough. They dream of being good at different things, wanting to succeed at everything. But they always see other people as more successful, attractive, intelligent and talented than themselves. They often feel like failures and tend to believe that everyone else shares this view, whether it's true or not.

Trying to excel in life, to succeed, helps to block out insecurities, low self-esteem and anxieties about a developing body. The control of food and body weight, becomes an integral part of that controlling lifestyle, trying to get a grip on their weight, when so many things are not going the way they would like.

People who develop anorexia tend to be introverted, conscientious and well behaved. They're often perfectionists before they develop anorexia and may have obsessive personalities. Add unhappiness and the perceived inability to do anything about it, and you have a risk factor for anorexia.

Bulimia

Bulimia, or bulimia nervosa, is characterised by binge eating followed by self-induced vomiting, periods of starvation and/or purging with laxatives. It's often driven by a feeling of panic, when an individual feels they have lost control over their eating.

This pattern may develop from anorexia, or from an overly restrictive dietary regime. Hunger and depression can lead to binge behaviour. The vicious cycle brings about feelings of self-disgust and secretive behaviour, which can cause difficulty in social situations and tends to dominate daily life. Bulimics tend to be within the 'normal' range of weight.

The physical symptoms of bulimia might include:

- Repeated episodes of uncontrollable overeating: bingeing.
- Attempts to undo the effects of binge-eating by vomiting, laxative abuse, or using diuretics.
- Fasting to undo the effects of eating too much.
- Excessive exercising.
- Bloating, constipation and stomach pains.
- Use of appetite suppressants and other diet pills.
- Feeling out of control, helpless and lonely.
- Swollen salivary glands.

Bulimia is accompanied by chronic anxiety and feelings of guilt and depression. The behaviour makes the sufferer tired, emotional, secretive and deceptive. It carries a risk of dehydration, poor skin condition and menstrual disturbances. It's also common to develop a sore throat and dental problems, due to the erosion of tooth enamel caused by vomiting. Weight tends to fluctuate within the normal range, so the problem is not as outwardly obvious as anorexia.

However, like anorexics, bulimics also feel the need to achieve, and seek approval from other people. They're often riddled with self-doubt, often feeling inferior or not good enough. Insecurities make them feel poorly equipped to achieve their goals. They may have difficulty fitting in socially, have problems with the expectations of other people and feel unable to meet social demands.

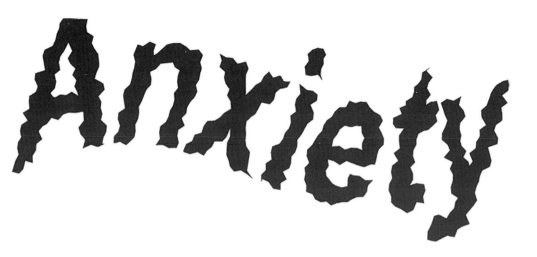

Stress, anxiety, hopelessness and depression, combined with loneliness and the absence of any way out, can culminate in binge-eating which releases tension – albeit a short-term fix. The desire to comfort eat spirals out of control. Then, purging the food eaten is a way of taking back control. Just as some people turn to alcohol or drugs to numb their pain, bulimics turn to food.

Like anorexics, bulimics can also be affected by exhaustion, starvation, abdominal cramps and discomfort, dizziness, swelling. poor circulation and sensitivity to the cold. Addressing the underlying problems and introducing healthier eating habits, are important parts of recovery.

Bulimia most often begins at around the ages of 16 or 17 in the UK, although in the USA, the average age of onset has dropped as low as age 12. However, bulimia can affect people of all ages. They usually share many of the same insecurities as anorexics and may have an unduly low opinion of themselves. Also see binge eating disorder, next.

Binge Eating Disorder

Binge Eating Disorder is characterised by emotional overeating with urgency. Sufferers eat more than they need, not because they're hungry, but in response to negative emotions. Binge eating disorder is faster and more urgent than comfort eating, which is more widespread. Emotional overeating becomes binge eating disorder when it's happening regularly, is furiously paced and feels out of control, causing weight gain, self-esteem issues and increasing dissatisfaction with body image.

The emotional hunger seen in binge eating disorder is characterised by:

- A sudden and urgent desire to eat.
- A demand for instant gratification.
- A focus on high carbohydrate, fatty and sugary foods.
- Still not being satisfied when the stomach is full.
- Feelings of guilt and shame.

Someone with binge eating disorder might binge regularly, eating too much food, in response to emotional problems. As with bulimia, they feel disgusted with themselves, and do it in secret, but they don't attempt to purge the food from their bodies after consuming it. The disorder is characterised by an obsession with food and often causes self-loathing and considerable distress.

Binge eaters eat until they're bursting, but still don't feel satisfied. They are not physically hungry and they feel embarrassed about their food consumption, so tend to eat alone. Like the other eating disorders, this disorder is associated with low self-esteem, depression and anxiety. It affects males and females and is more common in adults than young people. Guilt, shame and isolation may be part of the problem. These people struggle with their own weight issues too.

People who binge, either with bulimia or binge eating disorder, often have these awful cravings and they feel totally out of control. The cravings can be unrelenting, always there, day and night, making it difficult to concentrate on anything. All they want to do is eat. It makes them want to avoid social situations for fear of losing control. Constantly fighting the cravings is extremely draining, so lapses are almost inevitable.

Physically, they're not bingeing because they're hungry. Any hunger is satisfied quickly, so a binge goes deeper than that. In fact, once they fill up, they start feeling bloated, but it doesn't satisfy the craving for sweet, fatty, carbohydrate-rich foods, which just won't go away. The fullness after a binge might create breathlessness or abdominal pain and be accompanied by a variety of digestive complaints.

The individual might try desperately to resist succumbing to the binge by trying to occupy their mind with something else, but they can't concentrate. It's really difficult not to give in to this craving when it grips you, because you struggle to focus on anything else.

Purging Disorder

Some new areas of study are beginning to gain attention, and one of these is 'purging disorder', which while not officially defined in mental health at the time of writing, describes individuals who feel panic and lose control after eating very small quantities of food. So they don't binge, but they do purge. Some might think that sounds like a symptom of anorexia, but not all those who purge are underweight, so researchers have defined it as a separate condition.

Scientists from Florida State University found that people with purging disorder had a significantly larger release of cholecystokinin, a hormone responsible for controlling feelings of fullness, than bulimic patients. They also felt more gastrointestinal distress relative to bulimic patients and the control group.

Chapter 3

Understanding Eating Disorders

Many people with eating disorders are preoccupied with food and body weight, almost to the exclusion of anything else. This can make it difficult to concentrate on, or care about, other things. For anorexia and bulimia, it's total immersion in their goal: weight loss, perhaps in pursuit of physical perfection, social acceptance, or just happiness. Some are simply blocking out their pain. Others are afraid of their body becoming sexually attractive and just want to slim it away.

Anorexics and bulimics are usually terrified of becoming fat, so life revolves around calories and controlling or avoiding food. It makes them secretive and socially isolated so that others don't notice the extent of their problem.

A focus on achieving bodily perfection, or getting thinner, can be all absorbing. This helps sufferers to block out traumatic feelings about failing relationships, to numb painful emotions and to avoid the anxiety about the lack of control they feel they have over their lives. This focus on controlling one small part of their lives, is often a last resort and a way of coping when all else has failed.

Although self-starvation might seem like a suicide attempt, anorexics don't usually want to die. They just want to cope better with living. They have a nagging belief and determination that they have to become thinner, partly because elements of western society admire thin women and self-control, while frowning upon over-indulgence and people who are overweight. Also, many people with eating disorders say they think they're fat and, in modern society, that's a dirty word. Men experience similar prejudices, with the added requirement to build muscle.

Some people might be completely overwhelmed by life's problems but they're in control of their bodies, so a perceived weight problem is something they feel they can resolve, even when everything else seems hopeless.

Also, some people who become obsessed about their weight have a lack of purpose in their lives. This can lead to a feeling of hopelessness, loneliness and depression. Weight loss gives them a purpose and the 'high' that accompanies success can be uplifting and encouraging. A feeling of temporary euphoria helps keep them motivated, but it doesn't last, so the goalposts keep moving as the individual tries to regain that sense of accomplishment. They drive themselves harder to get thinner and achieve more.

A sense of achievement can be a big driver for some people with eating disorders, who are often motivated by personal accomplishment and success. It can make them feel better about their life generally, but the feeling is temporary. The constant push to get thinner gets more difficult and becomes addictive. This results in purging behaviours and it can eventually lead to starvation.

One of the reasons people cling to their eating disorders is that they take over their lives, quashing the effect of other traumas and diverting attention away from other problems, which sufferers feel powerless to resolve. An inability to focus properly on anything but food, weight and how to avoid eating, means that they don't have to face up to other painful emotions. Eating disorders can help to cover up a multitude of problems and inner conflicts, over which the individual feels they have no control.

Personality traits

Anorexics were typically cooperative children, afraid to answer back or make a fuss. They grew up trying to please people and sometimes felt it was necessary to hide their own true feelings because other people wanted them to be happy, not sad.

Personality-wise, they tend to be less aggressive and more anxious than their siblings. They often worry about other people's expectations and fear rejection if they fail. While this is common among many people, anorexics in particular can become overwhelmed by these feelings.

When parents are demanding, expecting success from their child, but offering little in the way of emotional support, the child might feel valued for their achievements, but not loved as a person. Anorexia proves they can be disciplined and becomes their greatest achievement. Anorexia can also be an expression of inner conflicts between wanting independence and wanting to be looked after. These shouldn't be mutually exclusive, but the condition of anorexia, unconsciously, makes a statement that the individual is controlling their life (independent), even though their physical condition gives the message that they need care.

How a diet becomes an eating disorder

An eating disorder usually starts off as a diet, which escalates out of control and becomes an obsession. In modern society, dieting is normal, or even expected, as you 'shape up for summer' or 'lose those extra pounds after Christmas'.

Outside the realms of seasonal dieting, a more serious attempt to lose weight can often be triggered by hurtful remarks, anxiety about relationships, or significant life changes. You might become anxious about your appearance and self-conscious about how you come across to other people. The desire to look good triggers dieting behaviour.

Sometimes, the 'out of control' element just creeps up on you. One minute you're on a high because you've lost some weight and you're feeling good. Next minute, you're addicted to that high and can't think about anything else, except the next goal: getting thinner. And so it goes on.

As your stomach shrinks, you fill up more easily, hunger is held at bay more easily. You feel good.

So you've just cut down on the sweet things and reduced savouries a little, with the aim of losing a stone. For the first month, that goes well, but you get impatient. You miss chocolate, are fed up, and become frustrated and disillusioned. You're not done yet; your stomach still sticks out.

When you eventually lose that stone, you can barely see the difference in the mirror. You're disappointed. Hungry. That initial 'high' feeling feels like less of an achievement now. The goal is surpassed as you just focus on weight loss per se.

Lose the tummy, lose the thighs, you say to you yourself. Perhaps you just need some exercise to tone the muscles, but if you're not the sporty type, that won't compute. If you are, you might be doing exercise all your waking hours, but still want to lose weight.

Disappointed after reaching your weight goal and still feeling like a failure, you're fed up. You want to give up, or take a break, but you're afraid of ruining everything. You give yourself permission to eat a decent meal. Just the once. You've earned it. But the trouble is, your hunger signals are all messed up and your stomach's shrunk, so you fill up quickly. You feel like you've eaten more than you should and panic.

You're convinced you've ruined everything. Fed up and irritated by your lack of self-control, you have a drink to help settle the meal. It makes you feel more bloated. And now you have cravings, but one more chocolate biscuit doesn't make them go away.

This is often a trigger point for either a full-blown binge, a period of fasting and starvation, and/or an attempt at purgation, which might include self-induced vomiting, a diet pill or laxative abuse. Severe dieting and fasting can bring with it the urge to overeat and a feeling that you're increasingly out of control.

When you embark on a diet, you deliberately ignore your body's hunger cues. This eventually starts to mess up your hunger signals and confuses your body about the feeling of fullness. You might feel full very quickly, but not satisfied. This lack of satiation can be a real problem, eroding your resolve and increasing the risk of a binge.

For someone on the road to an eating disorder, food becomes something they fear, the act of eating riddled with guilt and anxiety. 'Not eating' however, is considered virtuous and is associated with self-control and achievement.

You'll start to see that there's quite a lot of overlap between the different eating disorders. It's easy to switch between periods of anorexia to bulimia and back again.

A binge and the vicious cycle

So, you're uncomfortable, the diet's ruined anyway and your cravings are driving you insane. A frenzied pattern of eating ensues. You're out of control. You know it's bad, but you just want to satisfy the cravings. You want them to stop. Food is consumed so hurriedly that it may be eaten uncooked or even frozen. The binge comprises almost entirely of high calorie, carbohydrate-rich foods such as sweets, chocolate, ice cream and bread, or fatty foods, like cheese.

You do it once. You purge. You vow never to do it again and go away from the kitchen, exhausted, disgusted and overwhelmed by it all. You get back on the diet the next day. A harsh one. Perhaps fast for a while. You obviously haven't been strict enough before.

So the cycle continues. One day, when your hunger pangs are crying out and you feel drained of energy, you'll think that a little extra food won't hurt. But 'a little' just whets the appetite and then the cravings come back. You get carried away with these insatiable cravings and you binge.

Some people with eating disorders have described a split personality, with a hidden persona taking over when they binge. It takes control and the compulsion to binge is so strong, that sometimes nothing can stop it. The vicious cycle seems unbreakable.

Even while they're bingeing, a sufferer will be revolted by their own actions but they're desperate to satisfy the cravings. They feel awful afterwards and dispose of the food in the quickest and most effective way possible. This is usually vomiting, although they may use excessive laxatives, diuretics, or fast. They may do them all.

Sometimes sufferers eat so much that their chest aches and the discomfort is overwhelming. The only quick way out is to be sick and they'll keep vomiting even when there's no more food to come out, choking up liquids and saliva. It's a reaction to the sheer panic of prospective weight gain when their life has been focussed on weight loss for so long.

Compulsive eaters (not bulimic or anorexic), will skip the purgation, but will still feel the shame. And they'll probably be doing the same thing again next week, and regretting it every time.

So having done all that, are the cravings finally satisfied? No, but they can't take any more. The cravings are impossible to ignore and the whole process is so exhausting, they just long for sleep afterwards.

The cravings lead to binges, the panic leads to purgation, and the cycle goes on. It can cause a lifetime of despair, when it becomes an obsessive nightmare and an addiction.

The buzz of a successful diet

Once you start dieting and see some success, you get a buzz and a drive to continue. Pleasure becomes an obsession, but the perfect body is still out of reach, so new targets are set for weight loss, and, through starvation, each is achieved in fairly short periods of time. How far can you go? Are you thin enough yet? It becomes a challenge.

Targets drop from eight stone, to seven, to six and so on. All the time you're fooled into thinking that your body is becoming closer and closer to perfection. Or perhaps the thinness makes you feel more empowered to cope with unhappiness in your life. You get skinnier and skinnier and watch that unsightly fat disappear. It's exhilarating, and drives you on. You're becoming more and more gaunt.

As someone with anorexia or bulimia, you see food as calories, calories as fat, and fat as flab – things that society has rigidly taught you to avoid because the result is ugly and unacceptable. You've lost so much weight, you're anorexic, but you still hate your skinny thighs because they appear to have 'fat' on them. Even your bony bottom and flat breasts are 'fat' – and don't even mention the tummy that won't go down. You become obsessed with getting rid of this 'fat' and in the process, you make yourself dangerously ill.

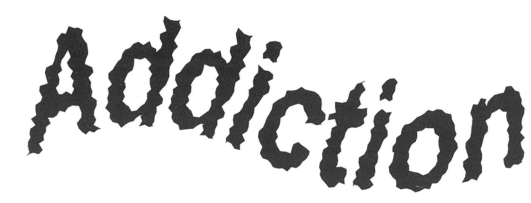

The addiction

Once a dieter has developed an eating disorder, it's very difficult to turn things around. They don't realise that they're addicted to the high of being thin, addicted to the numbing of their pain and addicted to the chemical cocktail that starvation creates, even when it's interspersed with bingeing and purging.

Eating disorders are unlike other addictions, because with drugs, for example, you can actively avoid your poison during and after recovery. Drug addicts can stop taking drugs with only temporary side effects; alcoholics can completely avoid alcohol; and smokers can stop buying cigarettes. Someone with an eating disorder however, has to learn to control their intake of food because simply avoiding it is not an option – if they don't eat, they die.

Fortunately, whatever your diagnosis, with inner strength and determination, you can still break free.

Case studies

Anna was bingeing and was sick as many as twenty times every day. The craving didn't subside from one day to the next and it became an addiction as expensive as heroin. She would spend £40 a day on food, which went literally, down the toilet. In a few frightful months, her weight veered violently from eight to thirteen stone and back again. As a child she was fed profusely by her parents as a reward for good behaviour. This was one of their ways of demonstrating their love for her. Unfortunately, it backfired – she put on weight and began dieting. Her weight became an obsession and Anna became bulimic.

Sophie was a very pretty child and as she grew up, her parents were very proud of her good looks, but they didn't seem to recognise her other qualities. Her self-esteem was dependent upon her appearance. Then at the age of 21, to please her boyfriend, Sophie joined him in midnight feasts of chocolate. After he'd gone, for fear of losing her figure, self-esteem, and boyfriend to obesity, she made herself throw up the night's consumption. After a time, he finished with her anyway but she had developed bulimic tendencies, which became an addiction that she couldn't give up.

Joanna Grenside, a 25-year-old PE teacher, became notorious in 1993, for wasting police time, and £20,000 of police resources, when she faked her own abduction in order to avoid the food and festivities that Christmas brought. Her disappearance triggered a police hunt, but she turned up at work two days later, looking muddy, dishevelled and claiming that she'd been abducted and held prisoner. It turned out that the claim was a hoax to avoid the Christmas festivities, where she knew there would be a terrifying amount of food and she wouldn't be able to control her compulsion to binge. During her disappearance, she had actually gone into hiding at Heathrow Airport! The court showed her leniency, and she went into treatment for her condition after the case.

Joanna's reaction to Christmas reflects how many people with eating disorders feel about the festive season. They are terrified of food because they feel that if they allow themselves something to eat, then they will not be able to stop. And fattening food is everywhere at Christmas, making it harder and harder to resist.

Some people with binge eating behaviour, see it as their punishment for living two different lives: One life is lived publicly, trying to look good, respectable and getting on in life, while the other is lived privately, in unhappy solitude, harbouring feelings of guilt and self-revulsion. As eating disorders settle in long term, sufferers often socialise less and move towards greater isolation, for fear of their private life being revealed.

Why diets so often fail

Researchers have shown time and time again that short-term diets are no substitute for a healthy lifestyle, which incorporates healthy food choices permanently.

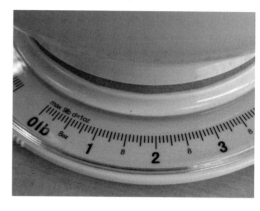

In one study, students were invited to eat as much ice cream as they liked. Some were on diets, others weren't. Some were given two glasses of milkshake to drink before eating the ice cream. Others were given one. Some didn't have any milkshakes at all. Among the non-dieters, those who'd consumed more milkshake, ate less ice cream. But among the dieters, the guilt of having indulged in their milkshakes paved the way for a big ice cream indulgence too. They felt that they'd ruined their diet, so they might as well make the most of the situation. The end result was that the dieters who'd drunk the most milkshake at the start, also ate the most ice cream. It's typical behaviour among dieters. After giving in to a single biscuit they feel such a failure that they think they might as well finish the entire packet. It's easy to see how diets can lead to eating disorders. Emotionally, food becomes more important to a dieter because they've been depriving themselves of it. So when a typical dieter gets upset they will break their diet and that will often lead to a binge.

Another study divided female volunteers into three groups. The first group went on a fairly strict diet, the second group followed an exercise programme, and the third group neither dieted, nor exercised. Five weeks later, they all sat down together to watch a stressful film and each had two bowls of nuts and sweets beside them. They were told to eat all that they wanted; by the end of the film, the dieters had eaten much more than the others.

When someone begins a diet, their body reacts by slowing their metabolism to preserve energy. It's a survival strategy against starvation. The extent of the slowdown is affected by how severely you diet, and this can lead to lethargy. According to a review of studies published in 2010, when you start to consume more, your metabolism remains 15 per cent slower than it was before you started dieting (*International Journal of Obesity*). On the upside, exercise boosts metabolism, so healthy levels of exercise are a good way of getting everything back to normal.

In 1944-45, thirty-six men volunteered to have their food restricted as part of The Great Starvation Experiment, instead of doing military service. They all began the experiment emotionally stable, consuming 3200 calories a day for the first twelve weeks, while they lived an active lifestyle, walking twenty-two miles per week.

Then their ration was cut to 1570 calories a day and they were told to continue living their active lifestyle. But as they lost weight they became increasingly tired, weak and complained that they felt old. They stopped caring about world affairs, developed mental apathy, lost interest in sex and were only interested in one thing; food. They became irritable, impatient and totally preoccupied with food. They were allowed unlimited chewing gum, black coffee, and water, so they consumed up to forty packets of chewing gum a day and fifteen cups of coffee.

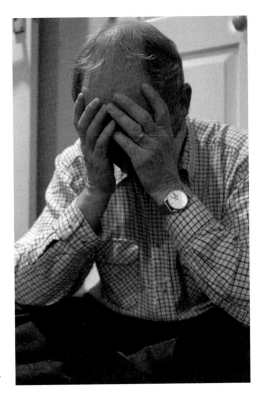

Then they started to 'cheat', eating foods when they went out. So a 'buddy' system was introduced, meaning they could only leave the lab with a chaperone, to stop them from cheating. Two of the men broke down before the end of the experiment. They were finding the side effects of starvation unbearable.

Their metabolism slowed, they became skeletal and their ankles, knees, and faces swelled. Some reported dizziness, sore muscles, coordination difficulties and tinnitus. The men started to see everyone else as fat, rather than themselves as skinny.

When the experimental period was over, some ate over eleven thousand calories per day and for many months they experienced cravings for food that they couldn't satisfy, regardless of how much they ate. The study began in November 1944, and ended in October 1945, eventually being published in 1950.

Increasing evidence shows that dieting is not a solution to weight concerns, but often results in weight gain. We will look at healthy eating in Chapter 11.

Chapter 4

Health Risks Associated with Eating Disorders

It's easy to assume that weight loss is a good thing, with no adverse consequences. Indeed, we're all taught that weight loss is beneficial to health. However, when you take weight loss to extremes, or use questionable methods, there can be serious consequences and it's important to be aware of them.

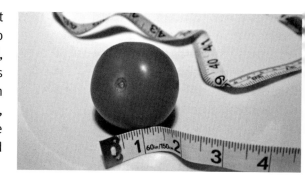

The short term consequences can include:

- A decreased heart rate, slowing metabolism, and low body temperature.
- Malnutrition, anaemia, fatigue and light headedness.
- Dehydration, poor skin condition, dry and brittle hair.
- In anorexia, the growth of fine downy hair on the face and neck is your body's attempt to keep warm while your metabolism slows.
- There is a risk of seizures among bulimics, which may involve loss of consciousness, involuntary jerky movements, and urinary incontinence.
- Barrett's Oesophagus is a disease affecting the lining of your oesophagus (food pipe), which may increase your risk of oesophageal cancer.
- Chronic Fatigue Syndrome may leave you feeling exhausted and unable to function.
- Vomiting may cause tiny red spots to appear around the eyes as a result of burst blood vessels, giving you an unhealthy, red and puffy facial appearance.

Yoyo dieting and weight gain

Some experts say that the regular fluctuations in weight caused by yo-yo dieting pose a far greater health risk than being overweight and stable. In 1991, a study in the *New England Journal of Medicine* reported that people whose weight fluctuated greatly over many years had a much higher risk of death, especially from heart disease, than people whose weights remained fairly stable. Furthermore, research tends to show that yoyo dieting will slow your metabolism, make you obsess about food and result in overeating and weight gain. These risks obviously apply with the weight fluctuations caused by bulimic behaviour and when someone is switching between bulimia and anorexia, as they constantly struggle with their obsession over weight.

Risks to your heart health

With anorexia, the body doesn't have enough carbohydrate for fuel, so it breaks down fat for energy. However, once you reach a very low weight, the body can start using muscle for fuel too. The heart is the largest muscle in the body, so this causes decreased cardiac mass, weakness in the heart, leading to complications such as cardiac arrhythmias, characterised by shortness of breath, chest pain, faintness, or loss of consciousness. Other possible outcomes include a decreased ability to engage in an active lifestyle, as well as an increased risk of heart failure and death.

Repeated purgation, common in bulimia, anorexia, and purging disorder, causes potassium levels to be depleted. This also increases the risk of cardiac arrhythmia, cardiac arrest and death.

Those people with binge eating disorder are also at an increased risk, because they'll usually have all the associated health risks of obesity, including high cholesterol, high blood pressure and an increased risk of stroke and heart disease.

The answer then, is not dieting, but learning to accept yourself, learning to overcome your eating disorder, selecting healthy foods and adopting a healthy lifestyle, rather than obsessing about weight. In the coming chapters I'll be trying to help you achieve all those things.

Renal complications

Purging, by laxative abuse or vomiting, causes dehydration, which can lead to renal (kidney) complications or renal failure. This can result in a build-up of toxic waste in the blood, because the kidneys are not working properly, and swelling of the ankles. Renal failure can be deadly.

Stomach ulcers

The linings of the oesophagus and stomach can be damaged by stomach acid among those people who regularly vomit to purge their food. Vomiting results in damage to the stomach and to the sphincter muscles at the entrance of the stomach. This can increase your risk of stomach ulcers and bleeding, which in extreme circumstances could be fatal. There is also a low risk of tearing the oesophagus or of rupturing the stomach.

Tooth decay and dental problems

Those people who vomit regularly are at an increased risk of acid erosion of tooth enamel caused by stomach acid. This will eventually lead to rotting teeth and other dental problems, as well as damaging your oesophagus. Vomiting can also cause hoarseness and recurrent throat infections.

Bowel complications

Eating disorders can result in constipation and incomplete emptying of the bowel, as well as a rare but potentially fatal condition called acute gastric dilation, following a binge, which causes upper abdominal pain, a distended abdomen and may require urgent surgery.

Laxative abuse can lead to other bowel problems, including pain and lazy bowel syndrome, with increased dependence on the aid of laxatives, enemas, or colonic hydrotherapy, just to defecate. Laxative abuse is dangerous for the cardiovascular system too, as it depletes essential minerals such as potassium, which are essential for a healthy heart.

Other digestive complications such as cramps, bloating, diarrhoea and incontinence may also present. Furthermore, eating disorders can cause a deficiency in digestive enzymes, which make it more difficult to digest food, causing additional digestive discomfort.

Osteoporosis

Most females with anorexia, or low-weight bulimia, either have irregular periods, or they've ceased menstruating altogether. This condition is called amenorrhea. Dramatic weight loss triggers a sequence of hormonal events, which result in loss of oestrogen from the ovaries, causing the cessation of menstruation.

Oestrogen is responsible for the normal menstrual cycle, and is also responsible for protecting the skeleton. Without it, the bones lose vital minerals, principally calcium, and become thinner, weakened, brittle, and liable to fracture. In short, the risk of osteoporosis in later life is increased.

Young adults up to the age of 30, are usually building up their skeleton, making it stronger so that they can withstand the losses that inevitably occur when they get older. During and after menopause, bone mass decreases, so building bone mass when you're young is important to prevent thinning and brittle bones when you're older.

However, when *young* women stop menstruating, they lose bone mass at a time when they should be building it, sometimes at significant levels that cannot be recovered when periods return. This raises their risk of osteoporosis later in life. There is also an increased risk of deformity and people with osteoporosis are at a higher risk of having a heart attack or stroke.

It is well known that high levels of exercise increase bone density, but even this is overridden by low levels of oestrogen if the woman is not menstruating. Therefore, the overall effect is still a reduction in the level of bone density. If a woman has not menstruated for up to a year, the osteoporosis may be reversible. Weight must be gained so that menstruation begins and plenty of minerals, especially calcium, consumed. After six years experts say that the trend probably can't be reversed. Therefore, the speculated cut off point is roughly three years, after which time it will be very difficult to recover the losses.

Men aren't exempt either. Men have a hormonal axis which among other things, is responsible for maintaining the integrity of the skeleton and this may theoretically be adversely affected when they're underweight and use up more energy than they consume.

Shock

Shock is a term for a deadly medical condition caused by a sudden drop in blood pressure. Failure of adequate blood flow to vital organs results in poor kidney function. It's common after serious injury, but can occur from hypotension associated with anorexia. Symptoms also tend to include hyperventilation, racing heart, clammy skin, anxiety and confusion.

Eye damage

A study published in the *British Journal of Ophthalmology* in 2010 showed that anorexia nervosa causes potentially serious eye damage. Parts of the eye (macula, retinal nerve layers and fovea) were thinner in women with anorexia, especially those who binged and purged. They said it was unclear whether the thinning, which was combined with decreased neurotransmitter activity, was an indication of progressive blindness or whether everything would revert back to normal when normal eating patterns were resumed.

The skin around the eyes can become puffy, red and inflamed when you vomit and it puts pressure onto this part of your face. Burst blood vessels around the eyes can cause an ugly appearance that takes weeks to clear – and if you're doing it regularly, will not clear. This can really knock your confidence, making you want to hide away, increasing your social isolation.

Fungal infections

Fungal infections, such as Candida Albicans, are another common side effect of eating disorders. Malnutrition can allow this aggressive fungus to overwhelm your immune system, taking up residence in your gut and undermining your health. The symptoms can include abdominal bloating, thrush, fungal nails, Chronic Fatigue Syndrome, aches, pains, bad breath, itchiness, soreness, a dry mouth and exhaustion. It can cause allergies and wreak havoc with your immune system.

Nutrient deficiencies

The lack of food consumed in anorexia and the process of purging can result in very low levels of essential nutrients and reduced immunity against illness and disease. Low potassium levels can result in muscle weakness and malaise, but the worst case scenario from low potassium is abnormal electrical conduction in the heart. This can lead to death. Malnutrition can also increase your risk of respiratory infections, visual impairments, heart attack and death.

Obesity and related complications

In addition to many of these risks, binge eaters face additional risks linked to obesity, including type 2 diabetes, stomach pain, joint pain, sleep apnoea and some cancers.

A shrinking brain

When you lose a massive amount of weight and are anorexic, your brain loses volume too. Fortunately, it recovers when you gain weight. A study by researchers based at the Columbia University Center for Eating Disorders in May 2010, showed that anorexics whose brains had lost volume, along with the rest of their body through the duration of the illness, can regain the brain volume when they regain weight. The research was published in the *International Journal of Eating Disorders*.

Death

The International Eating Disorder Referral Organization says that eating disorders can result in death from heart attack or failure, a collapsed lung, internal bleeding, a stroke, liver or kidney failure, pancreatitis, gastric rupture, or a perforated ulcer. Other risks include depression and suicide.

Beat, the UK's eating disorder charity, says that 20 per cent of those most seriously affected by eating disorders will die prematurely, either from the physical side-effects or from suicide.

Breaking free

These are just a few of the many complications you might face with an eating disorder. It really isn't worth risking your health in pursuit of a Western ideal of perfection.

I know that's easy to say, and that breaking free from an eating disorder is really hard. But hopefully, in the pages of this book, and with suitable support, you'll find the strength to break free.

Chapter 5

Our Cultural Emphasis on Body Image

It's no coincidence that eating disorders are most prevalent amongst young people. Ingrained in the heart of youth culture is popular music, fashion and contemporary imagery, which, to some extent, percolates throughout the whole of society.

Young people face enormous challenges and pressures. They often lack confidence and are worried about how they look to their peers. Relationships have huge importance at this time and social acceptance is usually vital to their happiness. They're forming their own identities, they may be looking for a partner and they're particularly susceptible to role models. Photographs of thin, elegant young women in glossy magazines, newspapers, billboards and online are unavoidable. Skinny women and muscular men, portrayed in popular media, are all part of the youth culture, in which many young people find themselves immersed.

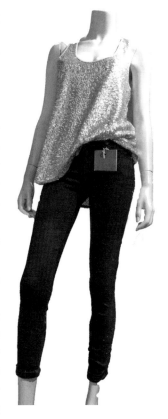

It's natural to place a lot of emphasis on appearance at that age – and at any age – because it's the first impression people get of you; it's fundamental to forming new relationships. Teens want to be popular among their peers and attractive to potential partners. Some have career aspirations that demand a good figure, such as modelling or dance. Some place more importance on body image than others.

Young people know that when they look good, they feel more confident, so working on their appearance can be an important part of building up their self-esteem. Music and youth culture often offers a fairly superficial outlook on life and many young people believe what the popular media tell them; fat is bad, thin is good – and variations on this theme. Fashion magazines carry pages and pages of adverts, suggesting that you need to buy products to fix your flawed appearance.

It's easy to get wrapped up in thinking that appearance matters hugely. Looking good is an important part of forming supportive peer relationships. So, as a young person watching your weight, you're just trying to fit in, be accepted and map out a positive future for yourself.

Many young people love the excitement and vibrancy of the fashion industry. They get sucked into the whole thing, including that anorexic 'ideal'. The industry does little to discourage the obsession with dangerously thin models, and in 2009 the supermodel Kate Moss, notoriously said, 'Nothing tastes as good as skinny feels.' It's a quote that's been bandied about on pro-anorexia websites ever since.

Being thin does make some people feel good. It gave me a boost in confidence. But there's thin, and then there's scrawny, and scrawny can become pretty unattractive as your weight falls lower and lower. There are better, healthier ways to feel good, boost your confidence and form healthy relationships, without needing to starve yourself or purge your food.

There is enormous pressure, especially among the young, to reach a physical ideal. I remember boys in my peer groups telling me I was too fat, too thin, too spotty, and too hairy because I didn't shave my thighs! I mean, who seriously shaves their thighs?! The girls were worse. They told me I was ugly, called me rubber lips, said I walked funny and called me 'pizza face'. I couldn't get away from school fast enough.

The fact is, many people do judge other people by their appearances and they expect their friends, peers and partners, to make the grade of physical attractiveness. They criticise those who fall short. So the pressure to conform to the Western ideal of beauty can feel huge and there's only so much you can do with spot creams and makeup.

Add to that the daily onslaught of criticism in some tabloid newspapers targeted at anyone who falls short of perfection, and the internet, with digitally enhanced images of muscular men and artificially slim women. There are images everywhere, giving vulnerable women and men, a feeling that they have a lot of work to do, to meet an ideal.

Fashion magazines and some aspirational lifestyle magazines, print images of anorexic women, to inspire their readers to strive for the same 'look'. These impressions encourage people to make derogatory assessments of themselves and of anyone else who doesn't match up. Many people aspire to emulate these images, which is why it's 'normal' to be on a diet, even among people who are a healthy weight to start with.

When you start to succeed at weight loss and people notice and compliment you, it can be motivational, increasing your self-esteem. People who look good are admired in our society and it helps them get great jobs, wealth and status. A slim figure is an attribute to be admired and you feel encouraged to continue. The thrill of the achievement is addictive and you don't want to stop.

How times have changed since the 1940s, when Marilyn Monroe boasted the ultimate figure; a healthy size 14. She had a figure that the media decided was the acceptable size at the time. Then in the 1960s, Twiggy came to stardom and media attention turned to her. The Twiggy image stuck, inspiring generations of supermodels, right up to the modern day. Fat, literally, became a dirty word.

Since then, society has taken the view that thinness is an attribute to be admired. It implies self-control and proper values. Obesity however, is considered to be unattractive and lazy, with other negative connotations. Some people are just sick and tired of feeling inferior and being judged. Even among those who aren't overweight, weight loss in pursuit of society's ideal, becomes a challenge.

Even employers can show prejudices. In the 1980s there was one department store who required their female staff to be between sizes ten and fourteen. Putting on too much weight was a sackable offence. I doubt employers would get away with that now.

Some parts of society educate us to believe that the views of others determine our worth. Society is definitely more liberal now than it was when I was growing up, but there's still a lot of pressure to conform. Many people seek the approval of others. It's natural, but they're constantly disappointed when they don't get it. And as much as praise can build up someone's self-esteem, constant denigration, ridicule, or being made to feel unattractive, can demolish it. Sometimes, it's unpleasantness from other people that can get us onto the downward spiral of the dieting treadmill.

It goes much deeper than vanity

It's easy to think that eating disorders are just about vanity, but they go much deeper than that. You might start off dieting because you're unhappy with your body and aspire to look more like the perfect people you see modelling products and clothes across media online and offline. But diets tend to leave you feeling hungry, obsessed with food and inclined to eat too much when you experience a moment of weakness. You then feel like a failure and it can be a vicious cycle.

When a diet becomes an eating disorder however, it's often being used as a coping mechanism for dealing with unresolved stress and trauma. The eating disorder is completely preoccupying, so it successfully distracts from seemingly impossible problems. While it may start out as an aspiration to look good, it turns into something quite different. For someone whose life has been characterised by bullying and abuse, total absorption in something achievement-oriented can be a welcome distraction from the other bad stuff. There's also an element of addiction, in terms of brain chemicals that make you feel good, and a longing to relive the buzz of accomplishment.

So it's not all about vanity. If pure vanity had been the problem, I'd have snapped out of it when my eye lids became red, puffy and inflamed, caused by burst blood vessels while vomiting. There was nothing attractive about that and I knew it. I was disgusted with myself and ashamed. This is not vanity.

For many sufferers, their body is often the only thing they feel they have any control over, so losing weight gives them the power they crave. Even if people show concern about the speed of weight loss or erratic eating patterns, it can be motivational, because someone who previously felt invisible is finally noticed.

Children with eating disorders

In the Western world, young children are now aware of modern demands for perfection. Even while I struggled with my own eating disorder in the 1990s, Great Ormond Street Hospital was seeing admissions increasing among children with eating disorders and it's a trend that has continued.

In school playgrounds, fat is the subject of cruel names and hurtful teasing. This abuse is hurled around from a very early age. One study showed that school children had a stronger aversion to being obese than they did to being physically disabled or blind. One of the consultants at the time, Doctor Brian Lask, who passed away in 2015, said that children were being exposed to sexualised images and the message that 'thin is good and fat is bad'. It was something, he said, that they were not ready for.

The average age of his young patients was 11, but children as young as 7 years old were admitted in severe stages of emaciation. Some suffered from such low blood pressure due to malnutrition, that they had gangrene in their feet. Some had lost half their body weight for their height and some of the girls' ovaries and other sexual organs had regressed to an infantile state. One 11-year-old he tried to treat could not stop vomiting. She ruptured a blood vessel in her oesophagus and died.

Today, children as young as 7 or 8 continue to be diagnosed, and Beat charity says they're aware of children as young as 6 being diagnosed with eating disorders, although diagnoses are patchy due to the lack of awareness of the disorders within this age group.

In 2013, Great Ormond Street hospital announced that a new study, led by the University College London Institute of Child Health had established that the number of people diagnosed with eating disorders increased by 15 per cent between 2000 and 2009. The majority of sufferers were adolescent girls aged 15–19, although males were substantially represented too with cases rising by 27 per cent in the same period. Males as young as ten years old were in the peak range for eating disorders unspecified (which means they don't fit neat definitions of anorexia or bulimia, but have similarities).

In recent years, the number of people with eating disorders has rocketed, with eating disorder related hospital admissions rising 8 per cent in 2014 compared to the previous year. About 1.6 million people are known to be affected by eating disorders in the UK, although it is difficult to get the figures accurate, due to the secretive characteristics of the illnesses, so the actual figure may be greater.

Young people are more likely to develop an eating disorder than older generations, although there are growing numbers with eating disorders among the middle aged and the elderly too. Motivations are perhaps different, but the remarkable rise in recent years across all ages and both sexes, suggests that, culturally, we still have a real problem. A US study conducted in 2012, among normal women over the age of 50, revealed that 3 per cent of female participants reported binge eating, 8 per cent admitted to purging, and over 70 per cent were trying to lose weight. Most participants said their weight had a negative impact on their life. Diet pills, excessive exercise, diuretics, laxatives and vomiting were all used as methods to control their weight and the vast majority said they were unhappy with their stomach. So the researchers concluded that eating disorders are not only the domain of the young, but they can affect women at all stages of their lives. Eating disorders are even seen in the elderly, where it can be quite perplexing, as their anorexia may be due to medications or complications relating to old age, rather than cultural pressures to be thin.

So why are more women affected than men? Well, everywhere you look we're surrounded by images of skinny models, used in advertising, on TV and in stores. Adverts and magazines are often intended to be aspirational, to make you buy beauty products, or keep you hooked on buying the magazine. Lifestyle websites and magazines aimed at women, carry these images alongside fitness plans and supposedly effortless diets that 'really work', topped off with tempting recipes for highly fattening desserts. It's confusing and contradictory; women are told that they ought to be as skinny as the models and should follow the diets, but they're also encouraged to eat the calorific desserts! As a result, many women are concerned, to some extent, about what they eat and many decide to diet.

Eating disorders are also now claiming an increasing number of men and boys, perhaps because in the past three decades there's been an explosion of idealised images of men's bodies all around us too. Popular entertainment on TV often encourages women to swoon at a man with a six pack, and if you walk into a department store, there are often images of a muscular man in whatever underpants they're selling. Now, men and boys are facing similar dilemmas and pressures to women. They aspire to be more attractive, slimmer and more muscular and it can become an obsession.

In one study, published by Manchester Metropolitan University, Senior Lecturer, Sarah Googan, and her colleagues examined how men respond to media portrayals. Men and women both assessed their level of self-esteem and their images of their own bodies on a questionnaire. Then they were shown pictures from fashion magazines and asked to do the test again. They all rated themselves less highly after seeing the pictures, showing that men are just as susceptible to media images as women.

Over-fifties with eating disorders

In 2012, the *International Journal of Eating Disorders* published a survey of US women over the age of 50 and their eating habits. Eating disorder symptoms, present at some point in the past five years, were identified in 13 per cent of respondents; 70 per cent said they were trying to lose weight; 62 per cent said that their weight or body shape impacted their life in negative ways.

When middle aged people suffer from eating disorders, there's an impact on their partners, children, work commitments and possibly on elderly parents too. They're potentially at a higher risk of negative health outcomes as their bodies are less resilient than those of younger people. Problems concerning the gastrointestinal tract, heart, bone strength and even dentistry can be more immediate and they're more likely to cause long-term damage in a middle-aged people.

Many middle-aged women are reluctant to tell their doctors that they have an eating disorder, because they feel that their doctor will think that they should have grown out of it. Imagine then, just how difficult it must be for men to talk to their doctors about an eating disorder, at middle age, or any age.

Elderly people with eating disorders

In 2013, *Today's Dietitian* reported an increasing prevalence of eating disorders among elderly people in the USA. They often go unnoticed because there are many potential causes of unintentional weight loss as you age, making it almost normal.

Causes of geriatric anorexia can be wide ranging, from altered taste to paranoid psychosis; from attention seeking behaviours to OCD; and from bereavement to dementia. Dental problems, and even prescribed medication, can lead to weight loss. If they feel out of control of their lives, then rejecting food gives them a feeling of control and can be used as a protest against carers. It's thought some cases of geriatric anorexia are attempts at suicide to escape depression and despair. Physically, they become prone to muscle wasting, frailty, poor immunity, depression and their risk of death increases.

Like their younger counterparts, elderly anorexics can be secretive and swear that they are heavier than they are. They refuse meals because they're not hungry or feel unwell. They may purge, with the elderly abusing laxatives more than vomiting.

Any medical problems that make it difficult for them to consume food need to be identified. Then any unresolved traumas need to be addressed with counselling, as well as help dealing with loss or bereavement, anger, lack of purpose, relationships, conflicts and low self-esteem.

Diet, medications and treatments should be reviewed by appropriate professionals and social engagement programmes put in place to get them more socially active and eating regular meals.

Chapter 6

Biological Causes

What causes eating disorders? Is it our individualistic and judgemental Western culture that makes people feel so bad that they're driven to desperate measures? Is it images in the media and pressure from peer groups? Or are there other factors at play? Well, although these factors do play a role, eating disorders are more complicated than that. Just about everyone is exposed to idealised images, but only a small proportion develop eating disorders. An individual's risk of developing an eating disorder can be affected by genetics, biology, psychological influences and environmental and social factors. When someone develops an eating disorder, usually a combination of risk factors can be identified.

Genetics and traits

If there's a history of eating disorders in the family, statistically, you're more likely to get one than if you come from a family without a history of eating disorders. Twin studies point towards genetics having a key role, although they're also keen to point out that environmental influences are part of the bigger picture. The family's attitude to food and weight may be passed down from generation to generation.

In April 2016, Columbia University Medical Center used a mouse model to study a genetic variant associated with anorexia and anxiety in humans. The genetic variant was given to adolescent mice, who were put on a calorie-restricted diet and placed in a stressful situation. The mice showed similar behaviours to human anorexics when genes, dietary restriction and stress were combined. This supports the theory that genes are a risk factor in the development of the disease.

However, it's not all genetic. Certain personality traits also appear to make an individual more susceptible to eating disorders. People who are prone to perfectionism, who tend to be obsessive and who are prone to negative mood states, are at a greater risk. Typically, people who develop eating disorders are sensitive souls who are anxious to be liked. They're usually good natured and are often willing to help others. They need to be appreciated.

In addition to that, some sufferers have long standing resentments, which can cause a lot of inner turmoil. They need to feel accepted and may take criticism to heart. Perfectionism may not be innate however. Some theorists say it's a reaction to not feeling unconditionally loved as a child, so the youngster defines their worth by their achievements and their ability to do things perfectly.

The characteristics of perfectionism applied to positive goals can result in healthy individuals who are successful at work. So these personality traits are not all bad per se, they're just misdirected. Being conscientious and concerned about doing a good job at work are desirable traits that can take you a long way in employment.

Chemical imbalances

There is a theory that people with eating disorders, especially bulimia nervosa, have lower levels of the neurotransmitter, serotonin, in their brain. This is a chemical associated with feelings of wellbeing and satiation. So low levels make it difficult to feel satisfied. One study showed that, even after a drug was administered to increase serotonin levels, bulimics had lower levels of increased serotonin than normal participants. Bulimics also binged more frequently when their serotonin levels were at their lowest.

The reverse is also true; high levels of serotonin cause appetite loss. In animal studies, where serotonin was released directly into the brain, the animals stopped eating, developing anorexia. Excessive levels of serotonin are correlated with a hyper, nervous, jittery feeling, which reflects an anorexic's typical behaviour of excessive exercise and hyperactivity. So it appears that imbalances in either direction could cause eating disorders.

Tryptophan is an amino acid (an element of protein) and a precursor to serotonin production, so when individuals start to restrict their diet, reducing their intake of tryptophan, this reduces their serotonin levels and can increase their risk of eating disorders. A study showed that when women consumed less tryptophan than their peers, they experienced lower moods, lower body image satisfaction and they felt out of control when eating. It might also explain why bulimics crave carbohydrate-rich foods; carbohydrates help tryptophan cross the blood-brain barrier, where it is converted first to 5-HTP and then to serotonin.

The Dopamine hypothesis

Some studies have indicated that people with eating disorders may have altered levels of dopamine, another feel good chemical. Dietary restriction has been associated with reduced dopamine levels in the brain, although evidence suggests the levels do increase when weight is restored. Low dopamine levels are therefore an effect of dietary restriction, rather than a cause of eating disorders. However, dopamine deficiency symptoms include sugar cravings, as experienced in bulimia, and apathy, which may have significance for anorexia. Rodents with dopamine deficiency starved to death because they lacked the motivation to eat.

In May 2012, the University of Colorado School of Medicine published a study in the journal *Neuropsychopharmacology*, which showed that the brain's reward centres are sensitized in anorexic women and desensitized in obese women. MRI scans showed that unexpected sweet-tasting solutions activated the dopamine-related reward systems of anorexic patients, but among obese individuals, the reward systems were diminished. This means that anorexics appear to be more easily satisfied by sweet foods than obese individuals. So anorexics stop eating and obese people carry on.

Another study, published in May 2011 by the University of California, showed that healthy women experienced extreme pleasure from taking amphetamines, which release dopamine in the brain's reward centre. But anorexics experienced anxiety when they took amphetamines, not pleasure. The researchers theorised then, that dopamine makes anorexics anxious, rather than experiencing pleasure. This would explain why they avoid eating food – it triggers a dopamine release, accompanied by feelings of anxiety, rather than pleasure. Importantly, the study was conducted with people who had recovered from anorexia at least a year earlier, so could not be attributed to something that occurs in people of a very low weight.

So does dopamine make anorexics feel satisfied or anxious? Perhaps both, or perhaps it varies by individual. Some anorexics seem to be quickly satisfied by small amounts of food and anxious about eating any more.

In animal studies, rodents who lost a lot of weight received enhanced dopamine reward responses in the brain. The researchers concluded that this showed dopamine played a role in appetite and weight regulation. It seems the exact nature of dopamine's role in appetite and weight, may be debated for some time to come.

Addiction to brain chemicals

When someone has consistently restricted their food intake, especially to the point of starvation, a feeling of euphoria is produced, which makes it addictive, say authors Duker and Slade in their book, *Anorexia Nervosa and Bulimia: How to Help*. The body releases adrenaline in response to 'hunger stress' which provides a burst of energy, and triggers the brain to secrete endokinins. These are chemically similar to morphine, with similar tranquillising and euphoric effects. Also, metabolites like ketones, which break down fat in the body for fuel when dietary carbohydrates are short, can result in a light headed experience.

Combine these experiences with the release of endorphins, serotonin and adrenaline during strenuous exercise – common among some anorexics – and the person with an eating disorder can become hooked on a concoction of pleasurable brain chemicals.

Is this a cause or effect of anorexia? The effect is more pronounced when the eating disorder has taken hold. However, very strict dieting and exercise could start the process, so that it escalates and becomes a serious problem.

Messed up hunger signals

Some researchers have suggested that anorexics cannot identify hunger pangs, so they don't know when they are hungry. They therefore don't eat when they need to and not eating becomes a habit which is hard to break. People who suffer from bulimia, binge eating disorder, or other erratic eating behaviours, may experience similar problems with their hunger cues, which seem all messed up. Sometimes they're not hungry. Other times they just can't feel satisfied, no matter how much they eat. They have to force themselves to sit and eat three meals a day, to get any semblance of normality, but this can be hard when your hunger signals are awry. Perhaps you're fighting cravings all day, or you're just not interested in food because your stomach has shrunk and you feel full. Also, if you're frightened of losing control, sometimes it might seem easier to avoid food altogether, but this just perpetuates the problem.

In June 2013, the University of California published a report in the *American Journal of Psychiatry*, showing that twenty-eight women who had recovered from anorexia or bulimia nervosa had elevated responses to the taste of sugar in the right anterior insula – a part of the brain associated with pleasure and addiction – compared to the control group. They suggested that inaccurate recognition of hunger signals or an exaggerated perception of hunger signals could increase the risk of eating disorders and suggested that developing treatments to enhance insula activity in anorexics, or reduce it in bulimics, could be beneficial. They added that anorexics with an overly active satiety signal in foods they enjoy, might respond to feeding with bland or slightly aversive foods, to prevent the brain's over-stimulation.

As far back as the 1970s and '80s, researchers found the hypothalamus (in the brain) has a role in the regulation of body weight. Damage to the hypothalamus can cause massive appetite and weight changes in animal studies, causing under-eating or over-eating. They showed that if the ventromedial hypothalamus is damaged, it results in the animal over-eating, because the ventromedial hypothalamus is what usually stops eating by providing a feeling of satiety. If it is damaged, then satiety is not experienced and the person becomes obese or bulimic.

Conversely, if the lateral hypothalamus is damaged, then the trigger to start eating is compromised, as this is a key role in hunger. The result could be anorexia.

More recently, in October 2014, researchers suggested that higher than normal levels of a certain protein could cause disruption to hunger and satiety cues. A study published in the journal *Translational Psychiatry*, reported that a protein had been identified, which mimics the satiety hormone (melanotropin). It's produced by certain bacteria, including Escherichia coli, and others that are normally present in the gut. The body produces antibodies (immune system responses) against the protein and among a group of eating disordered patients, the researchers found that blood levels of antibodies to the protein were higher than normal. These antibodies bind to the satiety hormone modifying its effect, which means anorexics feel satisfied too quickly and bulimics struggle to feel satisfied at all.

Food and sugar addiction

In July 2013, researchers from Boston Children's Hospital used brain imaging techniques to show that highly processed carbohydrates stimulate parts of the brain involved in reward and cravings, in turn, promoting hunger and overeating.

Overweight men consumed one low GI meal (where glucose is released into the blood stream slowly) and one high GI meal (causing a blood sugar spike). They were assessed four hours after each meal and the high GI meal resulted in less glucose in their blood than the low GI Meal. They also felt more hungry.

Put simply, this means that meals containing lots of refined carbohydrates, such as sugar and white bread, provided less energy and made them more hungry. The fall in their blood sugar levels also activated part of the brain associated with addiction, called the nucleus accumbens, which made them want more food. The researchers felt that their study offered further evidence that food addiction is real.

Brain abnormalities

In March 2013, *Science Direct* published research showing that the distorted perception of body shape frequently reported by anorexics is caused by a weak neural connection in the brain. The researchers felt this might explain why some anorexics perceived themselves as fat, even when they were underweight.

Another study, published in August 2013 by the University of Colorado's School of Medicine, showed that some regions of the brain were larger than normal in teens with anorexia. Specifically, anorexics had a larger insula, a region that processes taste sensations and is involved in body perception. A larger insula might be involved in the illusion of fatness when someone is actually underweight, suggested the researchers.

The orbitofrontal cortex, which signals satiation, was also larger in anorexics than the control group. So the researchers suggested that satiation might be triggered prematurely in anorexics.

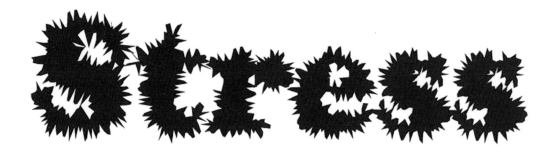

Chronic Stress

Stress can also trigger changes in the brain, which might lead to eating disorders. The stress hormone, cortisol, is released when people become stressed and chronically high cortisol levels have been seen in people with both anorexia and bulimia. Cortisol is part of the fight or flight response that has evolved over thousands of years, to enable us to escape from life-threatening situations. Cortisol inhibits appetite and may be part of the picture when stressful conditions lead to an eating disorder. But is stress the cause or the effect of eating disorders? There's no doubt that some people experience extreme stress and anxiety before an eating disorder grips them, but an eating disorder itself is stressful, so the situation can be self-perpetuating.

Complications at birth

The ABC of Eating Disorders, edited by Jane Morris, says that birth traumas and premature birth increases the risk of anorexia nervosa. Some people with anorexia nervosa have structural abnormalities in their brains, which can be seen using brain imaging techniques and it begs the question whether these abnormalities are present from birth.

Streptococcus bacteria

Anorexia has also been linked to exposure to streptococcus bacteria. Diagnosis of this bacterial infection in the throat often follows the presence of a number of other symptoms, most notably a streptococcal upper respiratory tract infection, fever and nasal discharge. PANDAS Syndrome is an acronym for 'pediatric autoimmune neuropsychiatric disorders associated with streptococcal infections'. Some PANDAS patients have exhibited symptoms of anorexia as well as symptoms of attention deficit hyperactivity disorder (ADHD), tics, and obsessive compulsive disorder (OCD).

Summing up

As you can see, there are many biological risk factors, but this doesn't mean eating disorders are inevitable, nor that if you've got one, you're doomed. There are also many environmental and social factors at play. It's often when many factors come together that disease develops. By tackling the disease from different perspectives, you can often overcome any biological predispositions and get well.

Chapter 7

Environmental Factors that Increase an Individual's Risk of Developing Eating Disorders

The people who develop eating disorders are often anxious, stressed and unhappy. Abuse and adversity are common back stories, more-so than in comparison groups. They have little self-esteem and what self-worth they do have, is frequently invested in how they look. Often their other problems become entangled with concerns over their appearance. Eating disorders are also sometimes associated with substance abuse, depression, self-harm and secondary diagnoses, such as personality disorders or OCD.

Family dynamics

Eating disorders are more common among adolescents because that's a time of change, of increased pressure, a time when they're forming their own identities, separate from that of their parents. It might be a time of conflict, if the parents don't want their children to forge their own path or make their own decisions (or if they don't agree with them) and it can be a time riddled with frustrating barriers and bitter disappointments.

Correlations have been found between eating disorders and problem families. Conflicts, aggression, ridicule and abuse can all impact on an individual's self-esteem and susceptibility to mental health problems. Atmospheres of fear and oppression can create an environment ripe for eating disorders to develop. A young person being neglected increases their risk of developing an eating disorder. Poor communication within families and burying issues and resentments by refusing to discuss them, in order to avoid conflict, is another risk factor.

In April 2013, the University of Warwick published an analysis of 70 studies involving more than 200,000 children and showed that negative parenting styles, including abuse, neglect, or even overprotection, made children more likely to be bullied by their peers than those who'd been raised with positive parenting styles. They were also more likely to become bullies themselves. Dysfunctional families, abuse and a history of being bullied are all risk factors for eating disorders.

Dictatorial parenting styles can leave a child feeling completely unable to control any aspect of their life and any attempt they make at control, decision making, or forging their own destiny is thwarted by their parents. Adult sufferers with dictatorial partners might feel the same. When everything else you try to do is thwarted and self-expression is punished, you feel completely suffocated and unable to change anything. Resentment builds up and the only thing you can control is what goes into your body. So feeling completely helpless in another aspects of life, can lead to controlling eating behaviours.

Another study published in April 2013, in the journal *Current Biology* reported that learnt helplessness results in depression, even in flies. Learnt helplessness is when someone, despite their greatest efforts, cannot do anything to change or control their circumstances – a common problem among children of problem families, because they can't just leave. The researchers said that when humans face impossible circumstances beyond their control, they would develop disorders, including eating disorders.

That's not to say that all the families of young people with eating disorders are bad, but this kind of environment certainly increases the risk.

PTSD

Post-traumatic stress disorder is something commonly linked to the armed forces and shell shock, but it also affects people in other walks of life who have recurring traumas relating to abuse, bullying, shattered dreams, bereavement or other issues. They might experience nightmares, repetitive memory churn, flashbacks and agitation. They might actively avoid reminders or triggers, be unable to remember important parts of the trauma due to blocking it out, harbour exaggerated negative beliefs and feel anger, guilt or shame. This can make it difficult to feel positive about anything.

Some people with PTSD discover that a focus on food and weight helps to block out their trauma. This is because eating disorders are completely absorbing, making it hard to think about anything except food and how to control your weight. The thoughts are unrelenting and merciless and that helps to block out other traumas.

Some people say that bingeing is like symbolically burying the negative emotion under a pile of food. Others may find comfort in eating.

Unrelenting Criticism

Pete Walker, a specialist in childhood trauma and complex PTSD, says that relentless criticism, especially from an angry or bitter parent, is so damaging to a child, that it can actually change the structure of that child's brain. Theoretical models say that this repeated expression of disappointment, anger and disdain are internalized by a child, who goes over and over the critique, forming an option of self-hatred and self-disgust. This starts to form part of their identity, affecting their thoughts, feelings and behaviours, until, eventually, they start to loathe themselves and lose the ability to nurture or stick up for themselves. The child's natural response to fight back has been destroyed through parental intimidation and threat of punishment.

Relentless negative reinforcement by a parent means this 'inner critic' dominates thought, often resulting in symptoms of PTSD. The individual is caught in a cycle of repetitive thought that drives shame and self-hate. Imperfection is seen as the cause, and they have a fear of abandonment, so they strive for perfectionism, which Pete says, is a defence mechanism for children who feel emotionally abandoned. Perfectionism provides meaning and direction for a child who feels powerless and has had little or no support, but because perfection is unattainable, they're prone to fail and the shame and fear are reinforced again.

Constant criticism can drive a lack of self-worth and a tendency towards perfectionism, because someone who's always felt criticised is always trying to be perfect, so they don't get criticised again. When they don't feel loved for who they *are*, they try to make things they *do* perfect. Then, they hope to be loved for what they *do*. Self-worth becomes tied up with achievement and perfectionism, which of course, can also drive the pursuit of a perfect body.

Abuse or neglect

Compared to wider society, a high number of people with eating disorders have suffered from child abuse or neglect. Estimates suggest that between 30 and 60 per cent of eating disordered patients may have experienced some kind of abuse, neglect, or trauma.

Sexual abuse makes children anxious about sexual development and maturity. They want to avoid further sexual experience by keeping their body small, infantile and unattractive. While sexual abuse is perhaps the most obvious and understandable risk factor for an eating disorder, physical violence and emotional abuse can also increase an individual's risk. Any kind of abuse can erode confidence and self-esteem, leading to a feeling of helplessness and despair. Food can help to relieve the feelings of tension, stress and hopelessness associated with abuse.

A study conducted by McMaster University in July 2012, published in the journal *Pediatrics*, said that psychological abuse, which makes a child feel worthless and unloved, is very harmful. Psychological abuse was defined as belittlement, exploitation, denigrating remarks, terrorizing a child, emotional unresponsiveness, or corrupting a child. It is associated with attachment disorders, developmental problems, difficulties with socialisation and fitting into society and disruptive behaviour. Eating disorders might be used as a coping mechanism.

The researcher was keen to point out that while telling a child to put their shoes on for the umpteenth time was not abuse, yelling at them every day, making them feel like a terrible person and wishing you'd never brought them into the world, is abuse.

Then in May 2013, a study published in the journal *Obesity*, said that women who had experienced physical or sexual abuse as children were considerably more likely to exhibit food addiction behaviours, such as bingeing, when they grow up, than their peers who were not abused. The researchers suggested that the stress of the painful memories caused overindulgence in comfort foods. Strategies for helping adult survivors of child abuse to reduce food addiction behaviours might include the development of early screening for trauma among women with a propensity towards uncontrolled eating, and the development of appropriate prevention programmes.

Depression and the effect of bullying

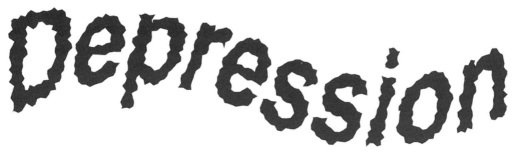

Depression is a key feature of people with eating disorders and they're often depressed from the outset, which affects their dieting behaviour, before the eating disorder takes hold.

Depression can happen for any number of reasons. Traumas can cause depression, as can failing relationships, divorce, bullying, insecurity and perceived failure in study or in work. Lack of purpose or a lack of things to keep you busy can also cause depression. Many people also say depression can be caused by chemical imbalances in the brain, so there's no outward cause for the condition. Controversially, this notion is being challenged by some psychologists, who argue that it's cheaper and more convenient to prescribe a drug than to get to the root of the problem. They say that depressive states actually create chemical changes in the brain, so 'chemical imbalances' are the effect of depression, not the cause.

At the risk of stating the obvious, depression can also be caused by other people being nasty. Some children become shamefully conscious of their body from a very early age – specifically 'the fat kid' at school, the one who could never get over the horse in PE. The National Centre for Eating Disorders says, 'Anything in childhood that dents a solid sense of self can lead to low self-worth, which is the root of an eating problem.' Low self-esteem and an innate sense of failure or inadequacy, can make an individual feel worthless.

Constant bullying is a terrible damage to self-esteem and some people have to endure it throughout their childhood and into adulthood. It destroys your confidence early on, leaving you feeling worthless by the time you reach working age. A child who is severely bullied at school may come to dislike themselves, and start to pursue bodily perfection, in search of peer acceptance.

Children feel particularly self-conscious when they reach adolescence and the pressure to look good can continue well into adulthood. Interestingly, anorexia is more common among the wealthy. Could that be because there's more pressure to look good, or thin, among the elite? Bulimia is equally prevalent across all economic groups.

In November 2015, researchers from Duke Medicine and the University of North Carolina School of Medicine, said that while it had long been known that victims of bullies were more likely to develop eating disorders, they'd discovered that bullies themselves are more likely to develop eating disorders too. The report published in the *International Journal of Eating Disorders* said that bullies had twice the risk of bulimic behaviours, such as bingeing and purging, compared to children who did not bully others.

Early puberty and sexual harassment

Early puberty increases a girl's risk of later developing an eating disorder, because her developing body is a source of huge embarrassment and no-one else in her peer group is in the same boat yet. So, unless she's popular and admired, she may become the butt of jokes, ridicule, and juvenile fun, which can make her want to shrink her growing body back into a childlike state.

In May 2013, Michigan State University published a study showing that sexual harassment increased concerns over weight and triggered disordered eating behaviour such as binge eating among women. The other interesting element of the study was that men were significantly more likely to purge when they experienced high levels of sexual harassment. It was the first such study to look at how men's eating habits changed in response to sexual harassment.

The pressure of change

The physical changes that take place during adolescence can take some getting used to and can be quite stressful. Peer pressure, identity formation and conflicts surrounding that, can all increase the risk of an eating disorder.

Adolescence is a time when many young people explore their sexual feelings for the first time. They may find aspects of this difficult, knowing there are certain expectations about body shape and they may be concerned about what potential partners will think of them. One study revealed that most cases of bulimia were associated with a young woman's first emotional or sexual relationship.

Hubert Lacey, professor of psychiatry at St. George's Eating Disorders Service in London, examined fifty female patients with bulimia, to determine the factors associated with the onset and maintenance of their disorder. He said, 'Bulimic patients describe a remarkably similar and consistent series of underlying factors, particularly centred on doubts concerning femininity but also including a poor relationship with parents, academic striving, parental marital conflict and poor peer group relationships. All patients described at least one, and usually two or three, major groups of life events; sexual conflicts, major changes in life circumstances, and loss.'

Confusion or ambivalence about sexuality may increase someone's risk of developing an eating disorder. In September 2015, Drexel University published a study showing that women who are bisexual or unsure of their sexuality have a higher risk of eating disorders than females who are either heterosexual or gay. Gay and bisexual men were also found to be more prone to eating disorders than heterosexual men. The male findings supported previous research. Results of female studies tend to be more mixed, but some of the increased risk might be related to anxieties around self-identity, or society's expectations.

Leaving school with an uncertain future can feel like a big pressure too, and it can be very stressful if your work or college options don't work out. Someone who leaves home for the first time may also be more susceptible to an eating disorder, because they are starting a new independent life, without the usual support network, or fall-back position of the family home.

Whether they're young or old, people who are going through significant changes or adjustments in their lives, tend to be more susceptible to eating disorders than people whose lives remain the same, especially if those changes are very stressful. So pressures such as divorce, bereavement, or depression may make someone more vulnerable to an eating disorder. This is seen among older people when they are widowed. The individual who is left feels lost, broken, and might lose their appetite and slip into anorexia.

In middle age, the kids leave home, there's the onset of the menopause, career changes and the potential for a midlife crisis. Have your hopes and dreams passed you by because life got in the way? It may not be too late to pursue them. Think positive. Depression can increase eating disorder risk, so it's important not to let negative thoughts sink into full-blown depression.

A study published in the *Journal of Clinical Nursing* in April 2012, identified triggers for eating disorders, which backed up previous research and clinical observations. Among the study group were people who had developed eating disorders after starting college for the first time, or those who'd developed eating problems following relationship changes, new jobs, hospitalisation, bereavement, or after experiencing abuse. The researchers concluded that life changes and lack of support were key triggers for eating disorders.

Western culture and our obsession with appearance

Western culture, which tends to promote individual achievement and success over and above collective values, traditionally has seen a greater incidence of eating disorders than Eastern cultures, which traditionally promote collective values. However, in recent years, Japan has seen an explosion in the numbers of people with eating disorders and some would say this is in part, because globalisation has meant that Western values have started to infiltrate Japanese culture.

Eating disorders usually begin with a diet, so even if you're just joining friends in a group effort to lose a few pounds, you increase your risk. Eating disorders can develop either from a change in the pattern of a diet, or a major stress event. Many bulimics had past problems with food, whether anorexia nervosa, obesity, a high-normal adolescent weight, or fluctuations in weight throughout their life.

In August 2012, research conducted at the University of Missouri found that among college students, appearance was considered to be more important than health. The young people they spoke to were more interested in counting calories than understanding the nutrition in their food. The researchers said that although participants realised images of fashion models in the media were digitally enhanced, it didn't stop them from wanting to achieve the same look, because they saw how society rewards women for looking good.

In March 2013, the *Journal of Eating Disorders* reported that male patients with anorexia nervosa associated themselves with feminine stereotypes and behaviours, while men with muscle dysmorphia were driven towards more masculine roles. The researchers from the Australian National University and University of Sydney, added that men are increasingly dissatisfied with their body image, and that trying to build muscle can be as unhealthy too, when they start abusing steroids, over-exercising and making unhealthy food choices.

Loneliness and isolation

In recovery from my own eating disorder, I found writing about my experience quite therapeutic. At the age of 19 I wrote, 'Modern lifestyles, expectations and requirements are forever becoming more demanding. As the high speed, hi-tech world around us carries on barbarically, heading in determined directions, everyone learns to grab, and look selfishly after "Number One". Companies and individuals mistreat, deceive and sue one another in immoral efforts to try and make sure that "Number One" comes out on top.

'Among all the formality, hustle and bustle of modern life, individuals get lost or disregarded. They feel unnoticed and uncared for as the world rushes callously by. They want to escape but there is nowhere to go. They need to talk but it seems that there is no-one to listen. Everybody's busy, too busy to listen and too busy too care. Troubled individuals become ever more isolated and distressed.'

This was how I felt. I was lonely, isolated, and very troubled. It was just my perspective at the time, and some may feel little has changed.

Loneliness and isolation can give you a bleak picture of the world. The Internet wasn't widely available in the early 1990s, and I'd never heard of it. Today, social media gives people a way to reach out for help that didn't exist before, but it's small comfort if you have no-one to turn to in the real world. Of course, social media can backfire if you get bullied online.

In the 1990s, information was relatively hard to come by and everything happened much more slowly. Today, we have instant access to information, forums and services that can help, which is a great step in the right direction.

However, the modern world also means we have digitally enhanced images of models everywhere, a thriving cosmetic surgery industry and increasing numbers of people both male and female, still worrying about their weight. If you're lonely and isolated, troubled and having difficulty integrating with society, it's hard not to think that perhaps it's your appearance that's part of the problem … and you might try to fix that.

Among older people, loneliness and isolation can lead to depression, apathy, and a corresponding loss of appetite, which might lead to anorexia. Often they don't have internet access, so they don't benefit from social connections online or the benefits of the information age.

A need for attention

Attention can be very comforting to someone who's feeling low. If you've been bullied, neglected, ignored, or felt invisible for a long time, then people complimenting you on your weight loss can give you an emotional boost and motivate you to keep going.

Dramatic or extreme weight loss gets attention for different reasons, but even that shows that someone cares and can be comforting. Everyone needs to feel valued by someone. Some people with eating disorders are so crippled by anxiety, loneliness and a need for approval, that even a little bit of attention can help.

So people should never criticise anyone else for seeking attention. It fulfils a basic human need. People with eating disorders often need support to get better. Initially, the attention that their eating disorder attracts may help an individual to cope with their circumstances, but in the long term, they'll need a helping hand to find other ways of coping with their problems and break free.

Perfectionism

I've said it before, but it's worth saying again that many people with eating disorders are perfectionists and are painfully meticulous in everything that they do. They tend to have an obsessive nature and when the two combine, you have someone obsessively trying to achieve bodily perfection – that is, their own distorted image of perfection.

People with eating disorders generally demand high levels of self-achievement and often believe that they don't look as good, or achieve as highly, as other people. They usually think that anything less than total success is utter failure and they judge themselves harshly against unobtainable standards. They rarely acknowledge it when they do well, because they can always see people who have done better than they have. Those who haven't done so well, aren't noticed.

In January 2013, the *Journal of Eating Disorders* published a study showing that people who are very concerned about body image come at it from two perspectives; the first is 'adaptive perfectionism', characterised by high standards for a perfect body; the second is 'maladaptive perfectionism' characterised by concern about what other people think of you and fear of making mistakes. The researchers suggested that the 'all or nothing' approach to perfectionism should be tackled, alongside how these individuals define their self-worth.

An earlier study, published in April 2009 by Dalhousie University, looked at why perfectionists tended to end up binge eating. They followed the daily activities of undergraduate students and found perfectionists most at risk of disordered eating are those who believe others are judging them negatively (as opposed to being self-critical). So a parent, peer or boss might be judging them poorly and they feel pressure to try to be perfect. This standard of perfection, of course, is far too high, and in the face of failure, they are more likely to binge than other students, as a way of escaping the feelings of failure, loneliness and depression.

Body dysmorphic disorder

Body dysmorphic disorder is where your perception of your body is untrue, such as believing you are fat, when you're not fat. Body dysmorphic disorder is more often considered a symptom of eating disorders, rather than being a cause, but if distorted perceptions were to take hold during the course of extreme dieting, this could lead to an eating disorder. There are degrees of distorted perception and, among bulimics in particular, there's sometimes a perception of 'feeling' fat, rather than thinking they 'look' fat. Sometimes, it's more about not being thin enough. Even among 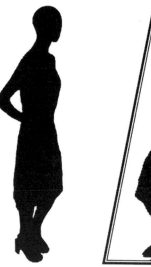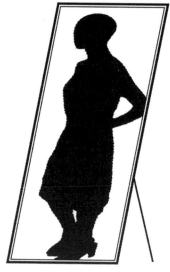 anorexics, some say they only tell the professionals that they believe they are 'fat' to offer an explanation and to protest against force feeding.

I didn't think body dysmorphic disorder applied to me until a woman at work, who I thought was slimmer than me, said she was on a diet. I was amazed. She was beautiful, but she said she was 'fatter' than me. This led me to compare my arms to hers, at which point I realised she was right. This thin girl, who I aspired to look like, was actually fatter than I was. I had a genuine misconception about how my body compared to hers.

In May 2013, a study published in the journal *PLOS ONE*, showed that anorexics who believed they were fat, unconsciously altered their body movements to allow for the perceived extra body size, when passing through a door.

The Highly Sensitive Person

Some people with eating disorders may be familiar with the phrase 'you're over sensitive'. People tell you to ignore nasty comments, bounce back and let life wash over you. However, not everyone finds that so easy.

Therapist, Elaine Anon, in her book *The Highly Sensitive Person*, explains that 15-20 per cent of people have a highly sensitive nervous system, which makes them experience physical and emotional sensations more strongly than the rest of the population. She calls these people 'Highly Sensitive Persons' or HSPs. These people have the capacity to do very well in life, because their sensitivity makes them think more deeply than non HSPs, analyse situations more thoroughly, assess all possible outcomes and respond with deep thought. They are the creative thinkers and the wise advisors, she says. However, their sensitivity also makes them feel things more deeply, so they are more affected by painful experiences than non-HSPs, who can just let it all wash over them. This may make HSPs less resilient to trauma than most people.

So HSPs who've had a traumatic childhood often struggle with anxiety, depression and other mental health issues. They typically have elevated stress levels and Elaine explains how having the stress hormone, cortisol, pumping around your body too much interferes with digestion, suppresses the immune system, causes insomnia and supports a worried hyper-alert mood state. This can lead to lower serotonin levels, leading to depression.

HSPs notice more of what is going on around them, process more information than most people and process it more deeply. It means they think things through more than average, might be more aware of subtleties in people's behaviour, and are more sensitive to physical sensations. People who are born this way can thrive in a supportive environment, but will often falter in an unsupportive environment, finding it more difficult to bounce back than people who don't absorb or process so much information. HSPs are more likely to struggle with PTSD in later life, following a traumatic childhood.

If you think you might be a highly sensitive person, you might find her book helpful. You might also be reassured to know that you're normal and that there are many other people out there, just like you. Support groups for HSPs exist in some areas.

Gut Dysbiosis or GAP Syndrome

A controversial theory about eating disorders has been put forward by Dr Campbell-McBride MD, in her book *Gut and Psychology Syndrome*. She believes that eating disorders are caused by abnormal microbes in the intestines. When the gut is home to too many nasty bacteria and yeasts, competing with the healthy bacteria for space, it's called gut dysbiosis. Dr Campbell-McBride says the resulting health problems can include autism, eating disorders, dyslexia, schizophrenia and many other conditions. She calls this effect Gut and Psychology Syndrome or GAPS.

Gut dysbiosis can be caused by antibiotics, poor diet, or even by not being breast-fed as a baby. She says many eating disordered patients are people who switched from eating meat to a nutritionally-deficient vegetarian diet, high in refined carbohydrates, like pasta, bread, pastries and cakes. These foods make people more prone to weight gain, so they get a hang up about their weight. Refined carbohydrates may also leave them depleted in nutrients, which means their immune system is less effective. They get infections and end up on multiple courses of antibiotics. The antibiotics wipe out their healthy bacteria, damaging their immune system further and destroying their gut flora.

She says Gut and Psychology Syndrome develops when abnormal gut flora, such as yeasts like Candida, start producing toxins, which enter the bloodstream. When the toxins enter the brain they can cause problems such as difficulty concentrating, distorted thinking and low mood. They can also affect behaviour and sensory perception.

The anorexic's altered sense of self-perception, says the Dr Campbell-McBride, is caused by this toxicity in the brain, which also affects their perception of social situations, relationships, what's important or trivial and other things affecting their daily life.

The abnormal gut flora also causes damage to the gut wall, which becomes porous, resulting in poor absorption of nutrients and digestive problems. She says that the high carbohydrate diet often given to these patients to 'feed them up', feeds the pathogenic microbes, so they produce more toxins, perpetuating the problem.

This is an interesting theory. I think other factors may have a bigger role in the development of an eating disorder – factors like low self-esteem and the family environment – but good nutrition is important and this could be a part of the puzzle for some people.

Obsessive weighing

In November 2015, Elsevier Health Sciences published a report saying that self-weighing may increase dissatisfaction with your body image, especially among teens. Researchers from the University of Minnesota recorded the self-weighing behaviours of nearly 2000 young people as part of Project EAT (Eating and Activity in Teens and Young Adults). They discovered that self-weighing activity was directly related to weight concern, depression, self-esteem issues and females' dissatisfaction with their bodies. The more they weighed themselves, the worse they felt.

A mixture of causes

More often than not, a mixture of risk factors combine before an eating disorder develops. They might be both biological and environmental, with some problems festering or developing for years. You might recognise some of these factors in your own life. Many people will experience hardships and bounce back without any obvious effects on their mental health, but when dozens of these factors come together, or you're hit by one or two in a really big way, it can trigger a mental health crisis or an eating disorder. For some readers there might not be any obvious background issues or answers here, but read on, because you might still find some helpful ideas in this book.

Overcoming an eating disorder is often a long, difficult struggle, but the feeling of freedom when your life is no longer controlled by your eating disorder is well worth the effort.

Chapter 8

Conventional Treatments

Many people who've had eating disorders for a long time are ambivalent about recovery. Their disorder has become ingrained in their identity and it's a focus for their lives, which might otherwise feel rather empty and lack direction. Or it might force them to face difficult problems they've been avoiding for years. Starting a new life, free from an eating disorder can be a frightening prospect, which involves overcoming their fear of food, reframing their sense of self, establishing new goals and priorities and getting back out into the society they've been avoiding, perhaps for years. The anxieties associated with an eating disorder don't just vanish either; during recovery, they have to learn to eat in front of other people, no matter how uncomfortable that feels, and resist the instinct to purge. All this, while having to face the demons of the past that enabled the eating disorder to become established in the first place. This can seem overwhelming and you need to harness all your strength of character to get through it. But you can. Every day, people are recovering from eating disorders, one small step at a time.

In terms of treatments available, there are many options, but initially, it might be worthwhile just finding out what your doctor can offer. There is no right or wrong answer in terms of treatment. Different people respond differently to therapies, so what works for one person, won't necessarily be the best approach for someone else. Recovery is a gradual process and your symptoms may change as you work your way through recovery.

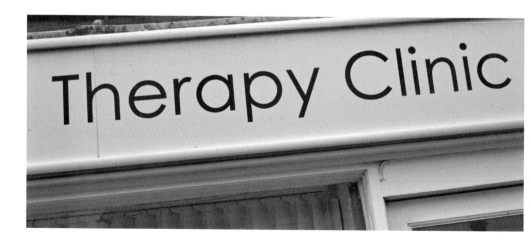

Psychotherapy

Psychotherapy is an umbrella term for many different types of therapy. The standard practice involves eating disordered patients talking to a therapist, either on their own, or as part of a group. They talk through their problems and feelings in depth, with the ultimate goal of reducing negative emotions, improving their outlook and overcoming specific mental health problems.

Art, music or drama can be used in psychotherapy too, and regular sessions can last for weeks, months or even years. Psychotherapy can help people develop the skills to cope with painful emotions and it's used to treat eating disorders, PTSD, depression, personality disorders, OCD and anxiety disorders.

Different types of psychotherapy adopt different theoretical underpinnings. The goal-centred theory says that misbehaviour is caused by unmet needs, so therapists should identify why people with eating disorders are motivated to behave the way they do; find out what needs are being met by the eating disorder that were not met before, then negotiate alternative ways for these needs to be met.

Some approaches to therapy advocate separating a child from their parents, when it appears that their parents may be a part of the problem. When a child grows up in an environment where their parents show little interest in the child's needs, instead demanding total compliance to parental controls, the youngster develops an identity based on over-compliance with authority figures and has little sense of their own needs and wishes.

They can then grow up with anxieties about parental separation as they reach young adulthood. They feel powerless and ill-equipped for independent thought, having spent their life trying to please authority figures. The conflict between their striving for independence and their separation anxiety, possibly accompanied by demands from parents who don't want them to follow their own path, causes great anxiety and a feeling of being out of control.

Extreme dieting gives the adolescent back some control – pursuit of thinness and control over their body and food intake provides reassurance, becoming entwined with their developing sense of identity.

Focal psychodynamic therapy

Among the most successful types of therapy, according to a study conducted in 2013, is focal psychodynamic therapy, a fairly new type of therapy, which aims to address the underlying causes of an eating disorder.

Focal psychodynamic therapy looks at how an eating disordered patient views food and the meaning of food for that individual. It then endeavours to explore new ways of coping with painful and distressing feelings, which are currently being numbed or suppressed by the eating disorder. By finding new ways of coping, the individual is able to let go of their obsession with food and weight and find healthier ways of managing their emotions.

There's a focus on preparing the patient for reintegration into daily life at the conclusion of therapy, which usually lasts for about forty sessions and obviously requires commitment and motivation from the patient, as well as a certain amount of endurance.

Access to focal dynamic therapy is limited in the UK and it is usually reserved for anorexics with other compounding factors, such as a personality disorder.

There's not a huge amount of scientific data for the success of focal dynamic therapy, but in October 2013, Heidelberg University Hospital compared the results of three types of therapy for the treatment of eating disorders, concluding that psychodynamic therapy and CBT had benefits over and above standard psychotherapy.

Seventy-five per cent of the anorexics treated in all three groups made significant weight gains following therapy, and the gains were sustained at follow up twelve months later. But focal psychodynamic therapy was considered to be the most successful method, because the patients in the other groups required additional inpatient treatment more frequently. However, the group receiving cognitive behavioural therapy saw the fastest weight gain.

Cognitive behavioural therapy

A close runner for second place, with a lot more scientific backing for its success, is cognitive behavioural therapy. This approach focuses on challenging negative thought patterns, to make you question what would really happen if you stepped outside your comfort zone and ate a whole apple, for example – or went a day without purging. In this way, it addresses irrational fears and behaviours.

Cognitive behavioural therapy challenges unhelpful attitudes about body and shape. It typically focuses first on changing patterns of eating and then on weight, shape and self-esteem issues. There's a focus on what might trigger episodes of unhealthy eating in the future and how to prevent a relapse.

By challenging the thoughts and fears that are stopping individuals from adopting healthy eating habits, cognitive behavioural therapy aims to normalise eating behaviour. This therapy also looks at social challenges the individual is facing, aiming to improve their problem-solving skills, breaking down overwhelming problems into smaller constituent parts, so that by the time therapy concludes, the patient is better equipped to deal with the challenges life throws at them. Patients are often given some homework to do between sessions.

Studies have shown that with the help of CBT, around 70 per cent of bulimics stop binging and purging, and in 50% per cent of bulimic patients, all symptoms are eliminated. Attitudes towards food are improved and dietary restraints are lifted.

In 2015, Oxford University announced a new type of CBT for people with eating disorders. It's called CBT-E or cognitive behavioural therapy enhanced, and it's a 'transdiagnostic model' which means that while, traditionally, CBT for eating disorders focused on bulimia and binge eating disorder, CBT-E can now be used to treat the full range of eating disorders. This is helpful, as many patients switch between the different disorders, at different stages of their illness.

All types of CBT focus on the present, not on traumas of the past. CBT is used in the UK for the treatment of stress and anxiety, eating disorders, PTSD and phobias. It's more widely available than most other talking therapies on the NHS and is considered to be among the most effective.

Psychoanalysis

Sigmund Freud's theory of psychoanalysis states that psychological illness stems from early deprivations and traumas. He also theorised that sexual repression underlay all mental illness. Weight loss was seen as a way to avoid sexual thoughts and feelings; something particularly relevant perhaps, to anyone trying to suppress traumatic memories of childhood sexual abuse.

Weight loss also reduces levels of sexual hormones in women with anorexia, which in turn, lowers their natural desire for intimacy. Many would argue this is the consequence of the disease, not the cause, but the two are clearly intertwined.

Based on psychoanalytic tradition, Hilde Brunch, a German-born American psychoanalyst, famous for her work with anorexics, suggested that someone with anorexia has an 'inadequate sense of self'. Someone who is socially and psychologically underdeveloped, due to a lack of confidence and assertiveness, will look for ways to express themselves. Restricted eating helps them express frustrations, insecurities and inadequacies. The psychoanalytic approach, therefore, endeavours to help the individual find their own voice and identity in a more healthy manner.

Psychoanalysis involves sessions with a therapist, who will ask what's on your mind at any moment, so they can explore the hidden meanings and patterns in your thoughts. This enables them to help you identify whether things that you do or say might be adding to your problems.

At the heart of modern psychoanalysis are the unconscious elements of the human psyche affecting individuals in ways we don't realise. For example, we don't always know where our fears come from, because the response is ingrained and automatic. But unconscious anxieties can thwart our potential and we may be hindering our own progress. Psychoanalysis endeavours to improve health and wellbeing by reducing psychological suffering.

Although psychoanalysis was originally developed by Sigmund Freud, his early ideas have been built upon over many years to create a diversity of different approaches now used in modern practice. In the UK, psychodynamic (psychoanalytic) psychotherapy may be available to eligible patients on the NHS.

Family therapy

The psychosomatic family process identified by Salvador Minuchin and colleagues, says that families are part of the problem when they're overprotective, rigid and refuse to address issues of conflict. This makes it difficult for a troubled child in the family to assert their needs.

The risk-taking needed for healthy adolescent development has not been allowed and conflict avoidance has thwarted all attempts the individual has made at independent thinking and behaviour. Rigidity in the family makes it difficult for a child to grow and adapt as they move into young adulthood, needing the freedom to express themselves.

Some psychoanalysts and family therapists working with eating disordered patients see a pathological family environment as the fundamental problem and will initially try to intervene to modify the family dynamics.

The Maudsley approach however, rejects this idea and says that the family is an integral and essential part of successful treatment. We'll look at the different types of family therapy below.

Structural family therapy

Structural family therapy attempts to alter the balance of power and break up inappropriate alliances, encouraging more support between children, promoting open communication. It endeavours to reduce a child's emotional reliance on the parents and to make the parents more effective.

If the family approach fails however, the therapists may remove the eating disordered individual from the family environment altogether, so that they can recover away from the influence of the pathological family.

There are organisations in the UK specialising in family therapy, but it's worth finding out if your doctor can refer you to an NHS specialist if you think this approach may be helpful.

The Maudsley approach to family-centred therapy

The Maudsley approach to family-centred therapy is different from structural family therapy. It rejects the idea that families and parents are pathological or responsible for the development of eating disorders, seeing the family's support as important in the treatment process.

Their approach to therapy is designed for adolescents with eating disorders and begins with an explanation of how serious eating disorders are, focusing on the dangers of severe malnutrition on growth and development. An environment designed to support improved eating behaviours is developed where the parents work with the therapist to re-feed and restore the adolescent's weight. The approach endeavours to engage parental understanding, love and support as an essential part of the recovery process.

Key features of the Maudsley approach are to restore weight and then hand control back to the adolescent, which happens when 95 per cent of the ideal weight is being maintained by the patient themselves. This is followed by discussion of normal development issues, to include those central to a healthy adolescence, personal autonomy and appropriate parental boundaries. It aims to establish a healthy identity for the young person.

A randomised clinical trial by the Maudsley Group found that family therapy was much more effective at treating anorexic patients with 90 per cent success rate, compared to 18 per cent success rate treating the individuals alone without their family present. This was due to the fact that unresolved problems within the family could be addressed after weight gain had been achieved, so that the patient did not return to the same environment, with the same unresolved problems that may have contributed to the development of their condition in the first place. Other studies suggest that between 60 and 85 per cent of family therapy treatments are successful among adolescent patients.

The treatment was developed at the Maudsley Hospital in London, so you might be able to get an NHS referral for this kind of treatment if you ask your GP.

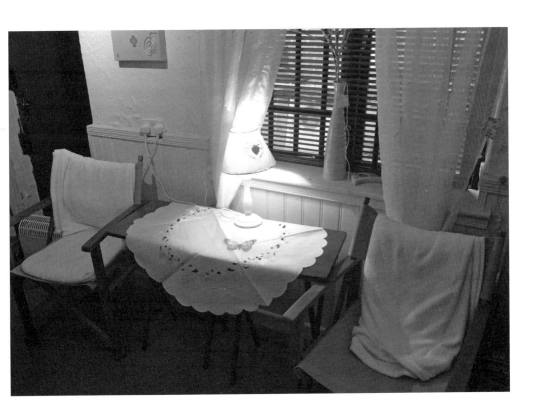

Psychodynamic therapy

Psychodynamic therapy focuses not on the eating disorder, but on the underlying issues that may have caused it. The approach is rooted in Freud's psychoanalysis, but it also takes elements of therapeutic practice from Carl Jung, Alfred Adler, Otto Rank and Melanie Klein. It aims to bring the unconscious into the conscious, with the view that the unconscious holds onto traumatic experiences that are too painful for the conscious mind to process. It's less intensive than psychoanalysis, focusing on immediate problems and quicker results.

In two trials at St George's Hospital in London, researchers reported very good outcomes for this type of therapy among a variety of age groups. If the patient is too starved to participate effectively, therapists will adjust their treatments to compensate.

In the UK, 'psychodynamic (psychoanalytic) psychotherapy' may be available to eligible patients on the NHS.

Ego-orientated individual therapy

Ego-orientated individual therapy (also called adolescent-based individual therapy) emphasizes assertiveness, autonomy and self-efficacy among its key principles. It involves an adolescent's parents in collateral meetings, to support their child's one-to-one treatment.

One of the fundamental theories surrounding eating disorders is that by focusing on controlling food and weight, traumatised individuals can avoid feeling the full force of their painful emotions. So this type of therapy aims to address the patient's fear of strong emotions, helping them to tolerate the strength of their feelings.

In a study, about two thirds of adolescents taking part befitted from this treatment, and while results were slower than with family therapy, they were as long-lasting at the one year follow up.

Interpersonal psychotherapy

Interpersonal psychotherapy looks at how relationship difficulties can trigger illness when conflicts and disputes occur, as well as looking at challenges like bereavement or relocation. This therapy aims to help the patient develop coping strategies to deal with the difficult feelings involved. For eating disorders, interpersonal psychotherapy tends to focus on interpersonal problems, such as family relationships and dynamics. Little attention is paid to eating habits or weight. It looks instead at solving the underlying problems and stressors that have caused the illness to develop in the first place. It's quite effective too, although studies suggest that CBT might be more effective. In the UK, interpersonal psychotherapy may be available to eligible patients on the NHS.

Cognitive analytical therapy

Cognitive analytical therapy uses techniques developed in psychodynamic psychotherapy and cognitive behavioural therapy to establish how a patient's behaviour may be contributing to their problems. Strategies for improving unhelpful behaviours are then explored using a mixture of experimentation and self-help techniques. This approach to therapy is theoretically available to eligible patients on of the NHS too, although different parts of the country differ in what's available.

Humanistic therapies

Humanistic therapies focus on self-development and encourage the patient to think positively about themselves and improve self-awareness. They help people to recognise their strengths, draw on their creativity, and explore their choices in the 'here and now'. A number of different approaches fall into the category of humanistic therapies:

- Existential therapy takes a philosophical approach to exploring the meaning of issues raised.
- Gestalt therapy looks at the individual's whole experience, including thoughts, emotions, and behaviours, aiming to make the patient more self-aware.
- Human Givens psychotherapy is quite new and it focuses on the innate needs required for wellbeing.
- Reality therapy is similar, in that it is based on the premise that the patient has not had their basic psychological needs met and that the eating disorder is a normal human response to that.
- Person-centred therapy focuses on an individual's sense of self-worth and whether they feel valued as a person. This therapy can help them towards greater self-acceptance.
- Solution-focused therapy is helpful to those with goals and a desire to change because it helps the individual understand their own strengths and draw on them to achieve their goals.
- Transactional analysis looks at how individuals communicate, and how this can be improved, by recognising the ego-states of parent, adult and child, which are within us all.
- Psychosynthesis looks at an individual's spiritual side and higher levels of consciousness.
- Finally, transpersonal psychology looks at the person deep within, peeling back appearances and culture, to explore the real person deep inside.

The types of humanistic therapies generally available to eligible patients on the NHS will be those focused on positive thoughts, self-awareness, strengths and opportunities.

Nutritional counselling

Nutritional counselling helps the individual to devise meal plans, agreed between the patient and the therapist. It can be met with resistance by eating disordered patients who believe their own perspectives on food are correct and don't want to hear them being challenged. This type of therapy is not as effective as family or individual therapy, but it can be a useful adjunct to other types of therapy; some would say that it's very important for eating disordered patients to gain a better understanding of nutrition.

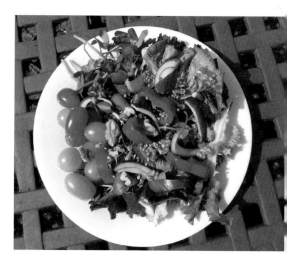

Nutritional counselling, or nutrition therapy, informs a patient about the components of a healthy diet, how many calories are needed every day to function and they can help a patient to plan healthy meals and snacks in a way that keeps the patient feeling in control.

This can help individuals to developed more balanced and healthy eating habits. On the NHS, a registered dietician usually takes this role. Privately, you can see a nutritionist, who may use slightly different approaches. Some other health professionals may have training in nutrition and be able to help. This approach is usually part of a broader treatment plan for an eating disorder.

Medication

Many people who develop eating disorders are suffering from anxiety and depression, so some of the medicines designed to relieve these symptoms can be helpful for people with eating disorders too. Based on scientific data, the most effective combination seems to be anti-depression medication combined with cognitive behavioural therapy for patients who are both eating disordered and depressed. CBT is often an effective treatment and antidepressant medication may be a useful addition if it's deemed suitable by your doctor. However, the medication has limited benefits and is not usually enough on its own. Take your doctor's advice on this, as they should be aware of the latest guidelines, preferred medications and best practice in this area.

Antipsychotic drugs are also sometimes used for anorexia when other treatments don't seem to be working. While mouse models on the antipsychotic, olanzapine, suggested this might be an effective strategy, there's little evidence of the drug's efficacy in human anorexics at the time of writing. In some patients, olanzapine may help to balance mood, reduce symptoms of depression and anxiety, improve cognitive function and slow metabolism, possibly causing weight gain.

A study by the University of Pittsburg in 2002, looked at anorexics treated with olanzapine. They saw reduced anxiety around food, less anxiety around weight gain, fewer obsessive thoughts and fears about being fat and they slept better. However, the medicine can also have some serious side-effects, which should be discussed with your prescribing doctor.

In studies, a variety of treatments have shown efficacy for patients with binge eating disorder, however, they may not all be used in standard practice. Antidepressants are used for their effect on normalising mood and reducing bingeing/purging behaviours. Antiepileptics have been studied for their effect of reducing binge eating behaviours in some patients, and some are effective weight loss agents, while a number of these drugs affect parts of the brain involved in the regulation of feeding behaviour.

Drugs used as appetite suppressants with satiety-enhancing properties have also been studied for the treatment of binge eating disorder, although this is controversial, and some have been removed from sale worldwide, due to safety concerns. Your doctor will advise you what treatments are appropriate and available, and it should always be remembered that medicines always come with the potential for unwanted side-effects.

Hospital inpatient admissions

Hospital admissions only occur in the most extreme cases of an eating disorder – usually when an anorexic has lost so much weight that their condition has become life-threatening. The patient is kept in hospital, either voluntarily, or they may be 'sectioned', which means they're admitted and detained in hospital compulsorily, in accordance with the Mental Health Act.

Inside a specialist eating disorders clinic, the focus will be on re-feeding, and putting an end to the destructive habits of purging and extreme exercising, so common among anorexics. Patients are put onto intensive treatment plans, with strict routines. Their daily schedule of activities might include one-to-one therapy and group therapy, as well as regular meals. The length of stay varies, and will depend on the individual's progress and weight gain.

These specialist centres are generally quite successful at re-feeding patients and restoring a healthy body weight. However, the downside is that many of those discharged face the same old problems when they're released. So they go right ahead and lose the weight again as soon as they've left hospital. One study found that 40 per cent of those discharged were readmitted at least once.

Treating associated mental health conditions

People who develop eating disorders sometimes have other mental health conditions, and taking these into account during therapy may improve the outcome of the treatment for the eating disorder. Associated conditions include:

- Obsessive compulsive disorder, which can be helped by cognitive behavioural therapy.
- Depression and anxiety disorders. The eating disorder itself creates a low mood, but many people were depressed and anxious before the eating disorder developed and might benefit from treatment. Talking therapies are thought to be more beneficial for treating depression in people with eating disorders, than antidepressants, which often have little effect.
- Personality disorders, such as Borderline Personality Disorder, which can cause unstable relationships and mood swings.
- Substance abuse is sometimes seen among people with eating disorders.

Getting better on your own

I recognise that some people might have trouble getting access to treatments. The NHS is oversubscribed with long waiting lists and people in other countries may not have health insurance or access to mental health services. So if you know you have an eating disorder, but your doctor won't take you seriously or refer you for specialist help, take heart – there are many people out there trying to get better on their own. You can find some of them in support groups and online forums, run by the eating disorders charity Beat.

I've heard about people who've been told by their doctor that they're not thin enough to qualify for eating disorder treatment; not suicidal enough to qualify for psychotherapy; or too troubled by traumas from the past to benefit from cognitive behavioural therapy, so they won't let them try it. Perhaps you've been told to 'pull yourself together' or 'snap out of it', or perhaps your disorder is so secret, no-one's even noticed – and you're scared to ask for help.

I've read about an eating disordered individual who deliberately lost more weight, just so that she qualified for treatment. This is an awful state of affairs. You may feel that an official diagnosis validates your suffering, but it's bad news for your health. I can only say, look elsewhere for help – there are charities and resources online. Talk to them and find out what help is available in your locality. Don't deliberately make yourself worse, just so that you can access services designed to help you get better.

See the chapter on complimentary therapies for free online therapies. See the chapter on nutrition to help you find a healthy diet that works for you and helps you relax around food. The chapter on recovery strategies (page 94) highlights approaches to recovery that you can embrace on your own.

There are some charities who will offer counselling free of charge to certain groups of people, such women who are pregnant. Other charities may charge as little as a fiver for a counselling session, so it's worth investigating. Many of the charities who offer counselling seem pretty pricey to me – they charge a day's wages for an hour's therapy – but search online and make lists of your options. Highlight the freebees and try to think positive! Surround yourself with people who make you feel good, and confide in a friend if you can. 'A problem shared is a problem halved' as they say. You'll find more practical advice as you work through this book, but for now, let's look at new and emerging treatments.

Chapter 9

New and Developmental Treatments

There are a number of treatments under development, from brain stimulation techniques to different types of talking therapies. CBT-E, mentioned in the last chapter, is a new and widely accepted treatment that is already in use, expanding upon traditional cognitive behavioural therapy, to offer an 'enhanced' therapy experience, helpful for anorexia and binge eating disorders. Many sufferers experience some overlap of symptoms during the course of their illnesses, so using a therapy that works for all eating disorders makes sense.

Other upcoming treatments include those designed to reduce anxiety around food and programmes designed to help prevent the onset of eating disorders in the first place.

New brain stimulation techniques under development

In March 2013, a study by Krembil Neuroscience Centre and the University Health Network was published in the *Lancet*. It showed that deep brain stimulation could be beneficial for patients suffering from anorexia nervosa. The method involves planting electrodes into the brain and it's already widely used for people with Parkinson's disease, Alzheimer's and obsessive compulsive disorder. Doctors tried the treatment on six anorexic patients in Canada and found that three of the patients were able to put on weight following the treatment. All other attempts to treat these patients had failed, so this was considered something of a breakthrough. It also improved the three successful patients' moods. Used in conjunction with other therapies, the researchers felt this approach had potential for the treatment of anorexia.

The downside was that the other three patients involved in the trial suffered from negative side-effects. One had a panic attack while the electrode was being implanted, one had a seizure two weeks into the experiment and a third found no improvements in weight or mood at the end of the nine-month study. So it doesn't work for everyone. The researchers hoped that their small study would lead to improved treatments for anorexia in the future.

Another study by researchers from Kings College London, published in March 2016, reported that a different treatment, using a non-invasive brain stimulation technique, reduced the symptoms of anorexia nervosa in just one session. The patients reported no longer wanting to restrict their food intake and no longer feeling fat. They also demonstrated improved decision making after the treatment. This treatment is called repetitive transcranial stimulation (rTMS) and it's already used to treat depression. It now looks like a promising treatment for anorexia.

Brain stimulation to treat binge eating disorder

In May 2016, researchers demonstrated that brain stimulation could have other uses in eating disorder treatment. A study published by the University of Alabama showed that sending a consistent low current of electricity to a specific region of the brain is an effective treatment for binge eating disorder. The treatment, called transcranial direct current stimulation (tDCS), decreased cravings significantly more than a placebo or 'sham'. The only side effects reported were a slight itching where the electrodes were located. The method has been proven to alleviate depression and improve the symptoms of Parkinson's disease and autism. However, this study was the first to demonstrate its efficacy as a treatment for binge eating disorder. It paves the way for further studies, testing the benefits of a series of tDCS sessions, which could introduce more permanent improvements. The researchers envisage the treatment working in conjunction with other proven therapies, such as CBT.

Developmental treatments to reduce anxiety around food

In April 2013, the University of California published a report explaining that anorexics experience extreme anxiety around food, which results in restricting their food intake, to reduce their anxiety. Their brain imaging research revealed abnormal brain alterations linking food with anxiety in anorexics.

The information has been used to develop new approaches to treatment, including 'psycho-education', which teaches patients how to cope with their anxiety more effectively. The researchers said that many patients were relieved to learn that their anxiety was related to how their brain was responding to food. It enabled them to look at ways of reducing anxiety around meal times, and develop a road map for effective treatment in the future.

Hormone to reduce focus on bodily flaws, negative emotions and anxiety

In 2013, Inje University in Seoul, South Korea, published a study showing that oxytocin, a hormone given medicinally as a nasal spray to anorexic patients, reduced their focus on images of food and fat body parts. A second study, conducted the following year, asked the same participants to look at people's facial expressions. After taking oxytocin, the anorexics were less likely to focus on faces of disgust and less likely to avoid angry faces.

Oxytocin is released naturally during pleasurable human bonding experiences. It lowers anxiety in social situations and is useful for people with autism. Prof Youl-Ri Kim, the lead researcher in these two studies, said: 'Our research shows that oxytocin reduces patients' unconscious tendencies to focus on food, body shape, and negative emotions such as disgust.'

Their research adds to the body of evidence supporting oxytocin as a treatment for mental illness and flags it as a possible treatment, specifically for anorexics.

Treatment to reduce the urge to binge

In June 2015, a study by Johns Hopkins University showed that the suppression of neurons in a certain region of the brain reduced the desire of rats to binge on food. The neurons in this largely unstudied part of the brain appear to be linked to external triggers causing overindulgence and addictive behaviour.

'External cues – anything from a glimpse of powder that looks like cocaine or the jingle of an ice cream truck – can trigger a relapse or binge eating,' said Jocelyn M. Richard, a Johns Hopkins University post-doctoral fellow in psychological and brain sciences and the report's lead author. 'Our findings show where in the brain this connection between environmental stimuli and the seeking of food or drugs is occurring.'

Rats trained to respond to an audio cue showed very high levels of neuron activity as soon as the trigger sound was played. They moved extra quickly to get the sugar available. The researchers found they could predict the speed of the rat's response, just by looking at 'how excited the neurons became' in this region of the brain.

'We were surprised to see such a high number of neurons showing such a big increase in activity as soon as the sound played,' Ms Richard said.

They used optogenetics to manipulate the cells using targeted beams of light. This temporarily suppressed the neurons, making the rats respond with much less haste, if indeed, they responded to the trigger at all. Being able to hold back or moderate the human response to binge-triggers could be a very useful treatment.

'We don't want to make it so that people don't want rewards,' Ms Richard said. 'We want to tone down the exaggerated motivation for rewards.'

Improving brain connectivity to help patients recognise perception errors

A study by the University of Illinois at Chicago in June 2016, used MRI scans to show that abnormalities in connectivity in regions of the brain responsible for insight, might go some way to explaining why some anorexics have difficulty recognising their eating habits as dangerous and dysfunctional. The same results occurred in individuals diagnosed with body dysmorphic disorder – common in anorexia. This lack of insight or recognition about their problem can lead to a poor response to treatment protocols.

Improved insight would enable anorexic patients to realise that even if they *feel* fat, they are actually way too thin. This would enable patients to reflect on those thoughts and feelings and make adaptive decisions to get healthy and recover. Without that insight, recovery can be much harder.

Long-term starvation affects the brain quite dramatically, so to prevent this impacting on the results, the researchers used anorexic participants who had since gained weight. They found that the regions of the brain called the 'caudal anterior cingulate' and the 'posterior cingulate' were poorly connected to the rest of the brain in anorexics, compared to healthy participants. Those who had worse insight scores showed the worst connectivity in these areas.

Abnormalities were also found in the reward and compulsion areas of the brain among anorexics and those with body dysmorphic disorder, which researchers said may be related to the rewarding feeling anorexics get from losing weight and compulsive exercising.

So what's the best treatment? The researchers suggested that new therapies could be developed to improve anorexics' ability to recognise the mismatch between their perceptions and reality. This might be achieved by using teaching methods that amplify the mismatch and using technologies such as virtual or augmented reality. Many anorexics can recognise other people with the disorder as being dangerously thin, but they cannot see it for themselves, so providing better visuals using these techniques might improve their recognition of the problem and support their recovery.

Behavioural Activation

For those who don't find CBT helpful, there is a new type of talking therapy, called Behavioural Activation. It focuses on helping people with depression to focus on how their behaviour affects their mood. It encourages people to seek out positive experiences and meaningful activities driven by their own values, helping them to find alternatives to unhelpful habits. This type of therapy can help lift depression, which is strongly associated with eating disorders. A study by the University of Exeter, published in July 2016, found that Behavioural Activation was as effective as CBT in treating the symptoms of depression. At the time of writing, it's not widely available, but studies such as this will help to pave the way for Behavioural Activation to be more widely used.

Drug to Inhibit Binge Eating Behaviour

In August 2016, researchers from the USDA/ARS Children's Nutrition Research Center at Baylor College of Medicine and Texas Children's Hospital, discovered that mice stopped exhibiting binge eating behaviour when a specific receptor – the serotonin 2C receptor – was activated. There's a drug currently used to treat obesity (a serotonin 2C agonist), which could replicate this effect in humans. The researchers showed that the serotonin 2C receptor, expressed by dopamine neurons, is important in suppressing binge eating behaviour.

Treatment for sugar addiction

A study published in January 2015, in the journal *Cell*, identified the specific neural pathway responsible for compulsive sugar consumption. The pathway from the lateral hypothalamus to the ventral tegmental area of the brain, when activated, increased the appetite for sugar among well-fed mice. Inhibition of the same pathway reduced the appetite for sugar, even among hungry mice, although they consumed the same amount of food. This suggests that the neural circuit controlling hunger behaviours is different to that controlling compulsion or addiction. This discovery could pave the way for drugs to be developed to treat sugar addiction.

New prevention programme alters body image perceptions

In December 2015, researchers from Oregon Research Institute published the results of a study, showing that an eating disorder prevention programme, called Body Project, alters perception of body image in vulnerable young people.

Young women at risk of developing an eating disorder were shown images of supermodels; a brain scan showed that a reward centre in their brains was activated by the images. After attending the Body Project programme, this reward centre was more activated by images of normal weight women, rather than thin models.

The Body Project programme involves young women in group discussions looking at the costs of pursuing the Western ideal of a super thin body. The method of questioning used in the programme is designed to stimulate critical thinking and ideas and to challenge some of the presumptions behind Western ideas of an ideal body image. The results have been very good so far, with three year follow ups showing the technique may be more effective than alternative prevention programmes.

After completing the programme, the young women valued normal weight women more highly than and had a lower opinion of the 'ideal' thin image. The programme is targeted at secondary school and college aged individuals, who are dissatisfied with their bodies and may be engaging in unhealthy weight control behaviours. The theory is that by critiquing the thin ideal in a supportive group setting, individual participants will reduce their support for the ultra-thin ideology, so feel less pressure to pursue it.

For more information and materials from the programme, visit the programme website: www.bodyprojectsupport.org

Chapter 10

Complementary Therapies

While conventional treatments are always considered to offer the greatest chance of success, some of these complementary therapies might help to relieve anxiety and improve the overall outcome of treatment for eating disorders. They're not scientifically proven, but anecdotally, complementary therapies are widely considered to be beneficial for their calming effects. They offer a supportive, attentive environment, which might be just what the patient needs at any given moment. Do check with your doctor before trying complementary therapies as an adjunct to conventional treatment, just in case they feel they would be detrimental to their own course of treatment.

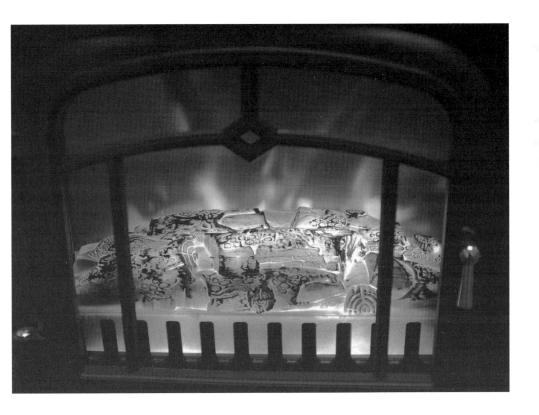

Mindfulness and meditation

Mindfulness is a buzz word that's very popular at the moment. It's all about living in the moment and experiencing the fullness of life. Mindfulness practice asks you to notice everything from the wind on your face to the rumbling of your tummy, to the smell of the grass and the sound of the bees. It promotes experiencing the fullness of taste and the subtle flavours in foods. It's about accepting what happens and letting it pass, not making judgements, not dwelling on thoughts, but just letting things come and go, pass you by, immersing yourself in that whole experience. Many people find mindfulness helpful and relaxing. However, it's not for everyone. There have been reports that it can make PTSD worse, by letting the mind wander free and enabling suppressed traumas to emerge, causing panic, or worsening depression. But there are also reports that it can be remarkably beneficial for people struggling with traumas.

Meditation and mindfulness are closely related. In meditation, you may try to focus on one thing: perhaps your own breathing, or another sound. Perhaps a guided audio. It's designed to relax you, reduce anxiety and alleviate stress. Many people swear by meditation to reduce stress and anxiety and some people swear that the meditation experience improves the more you practice. Not everyone finds it helpful, but there's something about sitting in the sunshine, feeling the warmth on your skin and completely immersing yourself in that experience, which can elicit moments of bliss. Listen to your instincts and do what feels right for you.

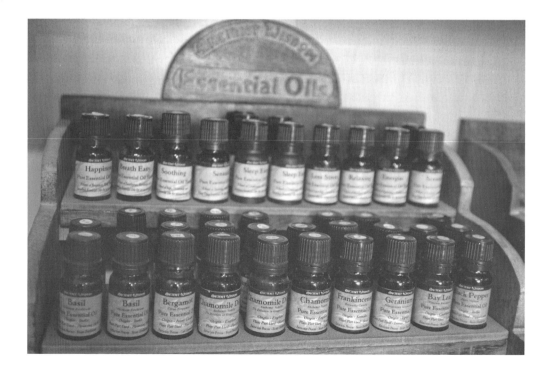

Massage and aromatherapy

Some people suggest that massage and aromatherapy might help people with eating disorders, perhaps by reducing their levels of anxiety. A massage is certainly a very relaxing treatment, which promotes good health, but all it can do for an eating disordered patient is to help them relax. That's great if relaxation is what you need. It's not a cure, but it might distract you from your troubles and create a peaceful state of mind, which is conducive to good mental health and emotional healing. Aromatherapy uses essential oils from plants to create a calming atmosphere. It's sometimes used in massage, or drops of oil are added to a relaxing bath.

Acupuncture

Acupuncture is a traditional Chinese therapy, where tiny needles are inserted into the body at 'meridian' points, to promote healing. There are acupuncture practitioners who claim to treat people with eating disorders, but evidence for its efficacy is sketchy at best. Even the British Acupuncture Council is reluctant to make any claims about their therapy's effectiveness in treating eating disorders. The only scientific study on this topic relates to a small pilot study undertaken in 2010, which suggested that acupuncture may improve quality of life, reducing anxiety and perfectionism among eating disordered patients. The participants were engaged in conventional therapy and using acupuncture as an adjunct to their treatment. It should not be used as the primary treatment for an eating disorder.

Acupuncture is a relaxing experience, like most complementary therapies. So it may make you feel nice and relaxed after treatment; less anxious, brighter, more chilled out perhaps – which could lead to the researchers' conclusions.

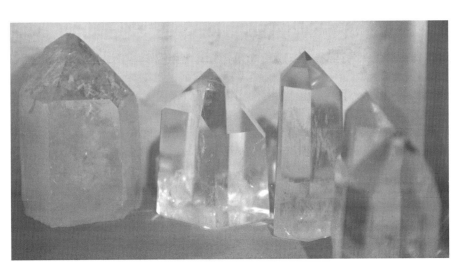

Free online therapies

Kooth is a free online support service for young people. Through their online chat service, you get help from friendly, qualified counsellors. www.kooth.com

SilverCloud is a service available through NHS referral, offering personalised programmes to help individuals with a range of mental health and behavioural problems, including eating disorders. Sign up to complete modules selected by your own online supporter. You can complete the modules at your own pace at times to suit you. www.nhs.uk/Conditions/online-mental-health-services/Pages/silvercloud.aspx

Futurelearn offers free mindfulness courses, delivered online. There are also courses about different aspects of psychology, mental health and anxiety, which might appeal, so take a look at the course listing. You engage with a supportive network of other learners while you're on FutureLearn courses, and there is no fee. www.futurelearn.com

Quantum K is a 'free healing experience' offering a colour and sound experience designed to promote harmony and wellbeing. www.quantumk.co.uk

Derek Chopra is a guru in alternative health and healing. He has a sample meditation available free on his website. www.chopracentermeditation.com

Living Life to the Full is a therapeutic website designed for people seeking to improve their emotional health. The course modules on the website are designed to promote good sleep, happiness and confidence, and you're invited to try sample modules for free at www.llttf.com

Headspace offers guided mindfulness and meditation sessions online. You can join free and take part in 'Take 10' – a free ten-day programme to find out whether this type of meditation appeals to you. Then, if you want to continue, you can subscribe to their other services. www.headspace.com

Enemas or colonic hydrotherapy

I suspect for some people, constipation exacerbates the eating disorder because it makes them feel fat and bloated, reinforcing the idea that they're fat and need to eat less, or purge. If this sounds like you, then bloating in your abdomen may be because you're constipated. If it's been a problem for a very long time, you may not even realise just how constipated you are. The obvious way to relieve the pressure of constipation on your abdomen is to get things moving. However, commercial laxatives are abused by people with eating disorders and regular use can cause lazy bowel syndrome, which just makes the problem worse. So the better solution is first to include more fibre in your diet, preferably soluble fibre, which draws water into the bowel, softening stools, helping move things along. Whole-wheat contains soluble fibre, although some people have digestive problems with wheat because it contains a lot of gluten. A better alternative then, might be fruit and vegetables, which contain a mix of fibres and often work better than grains in moving things along the digestive tract. Substantially increasing your intake of greens should get you moving. Regular exercise, plenty of fluids and a source of probiotics (healthy bacteria), such as live yogurts, in your diet may also help.

In some people with very stubborn constipation, increasing their fibre intake actually makes the constipation worse. In this situation, it's useful to know that consuming ground flaxseed with water, or taking flaxseed oil, can make it easier to 'go'.

When all else fails, enemas do the job quickly, even if the thought is a bit off-putting! Enemas involve popping a tube up your bottom and allowing water to enter your bowel slowly. This will loosen stubborn stools and enable you to 'go'. You usually lie on your right and let the water do its job for 10-15 minutes before sitting on the toilet and letting it all come out. Experts recommend a variety of techniques to make the most of your enema, from massaging your abdomen to remove faeces impacted on the bowel wall, to using fresh organic ground coffee to detoxify you, or adding probiotics to your enema. The latter is a popular way of ensuring healthy bacteria get moved in, while all the waste gets moved out! If you decide to try an enema, read the instructions that come with your enema kit thoroughly. Check online if you have questions about the process, and always oil the insertion instrument with olive oil or another oil, so that it slips in comfortably.

This won't cure your eating disorder, but finding a way to deal with constipation can help to remove the feeling that you're fat! Of course, if you're constipated just from lack of food passing through your system, then simply eating more food will help in the long run too. Do try substantially increasing the greens in your diet before embarking on more drastic measures, as this is usually very effective, and it's good for your all round health.

Colonic irrigation (or colonic hydrotherapy) is a similar therapy to enemas. It does the job for you, but it can be pricey and leave you feeling light headed.

Other therapies that may help

Other activities and therapies that have a reputation for reducing anxiety and promoting wellbeing are:

- yoga
- reflexology
- calm breathing exercises

- autogenic relaxation
- progressive muscle relaxation
- visualisation techniques
- tai chi
- hypnosis
- biofeedback
- music and art therapy

Use complementary therapies with your eyes open

Eating disorders are serious, potentially life-threatening illnesses, so don't put your faith in something too wishy washy, unless you understand that the benefit may be nothing more than a nice opportunity for a bit of pampering and indulgence, in a relaxing atmosphere, where everything is focused on you. These therapies are designed to make you feel good and they usually do. But there's a big difference between a nice relaxing experience and cure from a chronic disease.

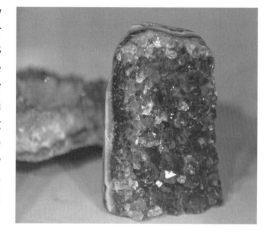

Chapter 11

Nutrition and Health

When I started dieting at the age of 16, it was a decision that eventually led to my eating disorder. I now wish I'd understood more about nutrition, because then I would have realised that I didn't need to diet at all. I just needed to tweak the foods I was eating. I was vegetarian, living on a diet, mostly, of pasta, cheese and chocolate. I thought I was eating

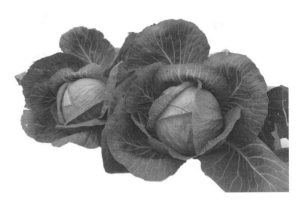

healthy foods, because they said, 'Healthy Eating' on the packet of pasta and sauce, dairy foods were rich in calcium and supposed to be healthy in moderation and I'd always have tomatoes or a salad with my savoury dish. I knew chocolate wasn't healthy, but I wasn't eating that much of the stuff. To be fair, I wasn't overweight either. But my tummy seemed huge. I looked down at it in disgust. Everywhere I looked, the media were on about flat stomachs and I felt like some kind of failure after my first boyfriend repeatedly told me I was fat and then dumped me. My best friend had a flat stomach – she was a totally different build – and I just felt unattractive and something of a pariah where boys were concerned. So I wanted to lose some weight.

I wish I'd known that switching from pasta to sliced cauliflower and onion with my sauce would have done the job. I could still have had my chocolate fix. I was a bit addicted to the texture of pasta and the satisfaction that comes from high-carbohydrate foods. Cauliflower isn't the same, but you get used to it. It would have been much healthier than calorie restriction, hunger, paranoia, obsession and eventual throwing up 'just the once'. I think we all said that the first time, before it got completely out of control.

So, getting a better appreciation of the effects that different foods have on the body can be quite helpful for someone who's worried about their weight. And understanding good nutrition can be a valuable adjunct to conventional therapies for the treatment of eating disorders.

By understanding how the body uses foods, you'll realise that you don't need to be so afraid of food. When I had my eating disorder, I knew nothing about nutrition and relied on the health claims on the packets, which rarely give the full picture. I knew in theory, that salad didn't make you fat, but in practice, by the time I'd become completely immersed in my eating disorder, I was terrified of all foods and even consuming a salad could send me into a state of obsessive panic, overcome with a compulsion to purge, for fear of being fat.

How can you get over this? Learn how different foods affect your body, and it'll help you find the courage and determination to test the theory that it's OK to eat. You'll probably be surprised the first time you eat something that you would normally worry and obsess about, you don't purge and nothing happens. You don't look like an elephant in the morning. It's actually OK. If you think you've gained a few pounds, you'd be wrong. It's usually water retention and will fall off in a week or so.

Good nutrition will help you emotionally too. It boosts your power of logical thought, can improve your mood and can help to stave off destructive thought patterns. A nutritionally enhanced programme of support will improve your cognitive functioning so that you're more susceptible to talking therapies and better able to help yourself.

But what's the right eating plan for you? Everyone is individual and I'd strongly recommend asking your doctor for a referral to a dietician, or seeing a nutritionist who can draw up a personalised plan to meet your own specific needs. Depending on your circumstances, you may need a different approach to another person with an eating disorder.

For example, if you're anorexic, by definition you're seriously underweight. This means further weight loss could be life-threatening; even maintaining your current low weight puts your life at risk. When a patient is at risk of death by starvation, feeding them high calorie meals is important so that they don't lose more weight and die. When your weight is dangerously low, gaining weight improves cognitive function, whether the foods you're eating are nutritionally dense or not, so there's a benefit to the mind simply from gaining a few pounds. However, there are nutritional deficiencies to correct too, so choosing nutritionally dense foods makes a lot of sense. Nutritional deficiencies mean you'll probably be suffering from poor immunity, fatigue, depression and poor cognitive function, so this is important to your overall wellbeing.

Zinc deficiency is common among anorexics – it's often a symptom of disordered eating, rather than a cause, but some people who have followed nutritionally poor diets before the onset of their disorder, may have had zinc deficiency from the outset. A study published in 1993 reported that zinc deficiencies in anorexia are rapidly reversible once the individual starts eating again, without taking supplements. More recent research however, suggests there may be a benefit in supplementing with zinc once a deficiency has been established. A study in 2006 found that zinc supplementation in anorexics resulted in a two-fold increase in body mass index, suggesting that it's an important nutrient to support recovery. Low zinc intake also adversely affects chemical messengers in the brain, which can lead to low mood. So zinc supplementation corrects these abnormalities, resulting in improved treatment outcomes. The researchers suggested that zinc supplementation should therefore be standard practice in patients with anorexia.

Other nutrients such as tryptophan, which controls appetite; essential fatty acids, which affect the mind; and B vitamins, may be supplemented for an initial boost against deficiencies as part of a re-feeding programme, but there is no alternative to a healthy balanced diet.

Some anorexics and people with a very low weight struggle to take in the number of calories necessary for recovery. In these cases, their health care providers may recommend liquid supplements to be taken with, or between, meals. They tend to be rich in protein and essential fatty acids and because they make you feel less full than solid foods, they reduce the amount of solid food that needs to be consumed and reduce the discomfort experienced after eating.

Juices, smoothies, protein drinks and meal replacement drinks like Complan might be helpful in these circumstances, but if you're so underweight that solid foods are posing a problem, you need specialist help and should consult your doctor for urgent personalised advice.

It's important to understand that eating disorders can kill you. Starvation can kill you. Never underestimate the damage you might be doing to your body and seek out the appropriate professional advice. There are people who can help.

Learning to eat again

Starting to eat normally is a huge and frightening step for anyone with an eating disorder. You'll no doubt be filled with anxiety about weight gain and calories, but if you're committed to getting well, and you're tired of your life being dominated by worries about food and weight, then you'll know that learning to eat more normally is essential to recovery. Part of that is accepting that if you're anorexic, a bit of weight gain is inevitable and, if you're bulimic, you shouldn't panic if you do gain some weight initially – it will fall off naturally when you embrace a healthy eating programme along with a healthy lifestyle.

Ultimately, the key to achieving a slim and healthy weight is choosing healthy foods. You can eat all the salad and green vegetables you want and you won't get fat. Binge on broccoli and tomatoes and you might feel bloated inside until they settle, but you won't get fat.

In pursuit of optimal health, I've had periods on a plant-based diet, and you'd be amazed how many greens you can pile high on your plate and consume without gaining weight. The key is choosing healthy foods. It's not about going hungry, deprivation, or worrying about whether you've eaten too much. Healthy foods will fill you up, but you need to learn to stop panicking when you feel full. It's OK to feel full, so fight the rising panic.

If you're strong enough to restrict your food and develop an eating disorder, you're strong enough to fight the fear of being full. The occasional overindulgence is nothing to worry about either. It happens. Food will go down. Four hours later, you won't feel fat. You might feel hungry again. That's normal. Embrace being normal. Cherish yourself.

Now, as I've said, there are foods like greens, that are really, *really* healthy and pose zero risk of you getting fat, regardless of how much you eat. I remember being so terrified of food that I once vomited after eating one tomato. That was all I'd eaten all day and I was starving, but I was also completely terrified of food and out of control. Frankly, that purging was stupid. A tomato wouldn't have made a bit of difference. Seriously, believe me, you can eat a whole tub of tomatoes and you won't get fat. You might feel full or even a bit bloated in the short term while you digest it, but you won't get fat.

So chill out and acknowledge that it's OK to eat some foods. Now let's go a step further. Those breads, cakes, pastries, and biscuits that you try to avoid because otherwise you want to binge on them? A bit of what you fancy won't make you fat either. So don't lose the plot if you give in and have a biscuit. It won't kill you – and importantly, it won't make you fat. Give yourself a break. If you have 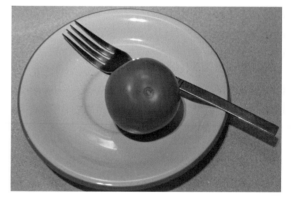 four or five, it doesn't matter. Don't purge. Don't fast. Just love yourself. As part of a healthy diet, it's OK to indulge sometimes. It won't make you fat. It's what you eat long-term that matters. Resist the urge to binge, 'because I ate three biscuits and have blown everything!' You haven't blown everything. Fight your instincts so that you can learn to eat healthily. And if you do binge, just accept that it happened and start again on a healthy eating programme the next day ... or the next meal time. It's OK. Don't beat yourself up. Your weight will stabilise when you're on a healthy eating programme; any ups and downs in the meantime should be ignored as part of the natural fluctuations that occur while you're in recovery. In fact, why don't you put the scales away and commit to stop weighing yourself every day?

Constant bingeing on breads, pastries and chocolates, obviously will add weight, so if you have an uncontrollable urge, binge on green vegetables. Go for it! Eat all that you want! Raw ideally. This is likely to curb your appetite for a binge. It won't satisfy your cravings for high carbohydrate foods, but bingeing on carbohydrates didn't satisfy them either did it? It just made you miserable. If you do binge on greens or tomatoes, then don't worry about it. It will go down in due course and it won't make you fat. You don't need to purge. Do remember though, that binging can lead to a ruptured stomach, which can be deadly. So when I say 'go for it', I mean fill up; feel free with those healthy foods. But don't binge so much that you rupture your stomach.

What if you're overweight already? Don't panic. Let's get your eating under control and get you onto a healthy eating programme. There's no need to diet. Diets are bad for weight loss, they play havoc with your metabolism and they make you unhappy. They tend to lead to eating disorders among those people who are most susceptible to them. Diets are bad news. If you get onto a healthy eating programme, then your weight will reach a healthy level naturally. You won't need to diet. It's just about choosing healthy foods and healthy living.

Nutritional therapy

NHS dieticians and private nutritionists work with individuals to develop personalised eating plans. If you get the offer of one-to-one support grab it and work with your therapist to develop an eating plan that suits you.

If you have safe foods that you're happy to eat, that's great. Are there others you could include? How about foods rich in zinc, essential fatty acids, and tryptophan – all nutrients linked to positive outcomes in eating disordered patients?

Essential fatty acids (EFA) aren't as scary as they sound. One important EFA is omega 3. This healthy oil can improve your mood, alleviate depression and assist weight loss. Did you get that? Consuming omega 3 oils can actually help you lose weight! Now, we don't want you to lose weight if you're anorexic already, but the omega 3 oils are still really beneficial for your good health – they improve your capacity for complex thought, make you feel happier, and boost your immune system. They will help you to break free from your eating disorder, by supporting your mind. Omega 3 can be found in oily fish, or, if you're vegetarian, good sources include flax seeds, walnuts, hemp seeds, hemp oil and soya products.

Foods rich in zinc enhance your thought processes and empower your mind. Nuts, seeds, red meat, lentils, beans, quinoa and shrimp are all good sources of zinc. Zinc supplements might help, but they're no substitute for good foods. Nuts and seeds are also good sources of omega 6, which is good for a healthy mind. Lentils and beans are low fat and nutritionally dense. These are healthy foods that won't make you fat and red meat is full of nutrients.

Protein-rich foods, such as meat, fish, nuts and seeds, are also associated with healthy weight control, and strong muscles. You must be fed up of feeling tired, weak and out of control. Deliberately adding some protein into your diet might improve muscle strength, support your mind and promote a healthy appetite.

Tryptophan is another nutrient found in protein rich foods, which is beneficial for the recovery of some eating disordered patients, because it boosts serotonin, a feel-good chemical in the brain and is thought to reduce the risk of binge eating behaviours.

What about breads and carbohydrates? Do you feel out of control around these foods? Don't panic. Having some carbohydrate in your diet is a good thing. Carbohydrates give you energy and make you feel good. This is probably why they're everyone's favourite binge food – they release pleasurable chemicals in the brain. If you're fed up of being tired, then carbohydrates are the fastest way of getting energy. But if you feel completely out of control around some carbohydrates, like grains, it's OK to focus on consuming other foods for now; fresh fruits and vegetables are good choices. Most foods contain some carbohydrate, so you'll get the energy you need.

Feel free with vegetables, beans and pulses. These will release energy slowly into your bloodstream so you feel less tired and more healthy.

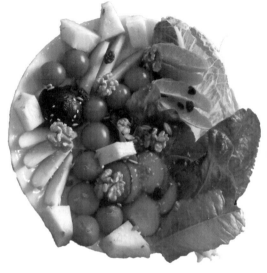

If you eat some pastries and feel out of control, don't panic. It's OK. You won't get fat if this is in the context of a healthy eating programme and a healthy lifestyle. Don't binge because you ate an oat cake – or even a whole packet. Sensible carbohydrate consumption will give you energy, not make you fat. If you're worried about carbohydrates, choose healthy carbohydrates – wholegrains and oat cakes, rather than refined flour, pasta and pizza. This way, you can be assured that what you're eating is good for your body and is healing. If you're underweight, it makes sense to include some complex carbohydrates into your healthy eating programme. You need them to avoid becoming dangerously low in weight and risking your life.

Healthy eating doesn't mean you can't have sweet foods. It just means your cupboards are stocked with healthier choices, so you can give yourself permission to eat and feel less worried about the consequences. You can still have treats, but hopefully, after a period of healthy eating, you won't want them all the time.

NHS guidelines say that a woman should eat around 2000 calories a day, and a man around 2500, to maintain a healthy body weight. This might seem a bit overwhelming if you've been worrying about calories in single figures. But the good news is that even if you're not comfortable eating that much initially, it gives you permission to eat more, without purging. Initially, as you care for your body and feed yourself healthy meals, you might still fall short of that figure if you're anxious about food. You might be surprised when you don't get fat. This will be reassuring and give you the confidence to continue.

If you have a moment of weakness and binge, you're probably still within the daily allowance, so don't panic. Many people find counting calories detrimental to recovery, so try not to obsess about it; if you go over, don't panic. Just let it go down. Start again the next day. Stick to your healthy eating programme most of the time and you'll get there.

The glycaemic index of foods

One thing I wish I'd understood when I was in recovery from an eating disorder is the glycaemic index of foods. It shows the impact on blood sugar of certain foods and can be a useful guide to healthy foods for blood sugar balance and weight control. Foods with a low GI are foods you can eat freely without worrying about blood sugar or weight. Foods with a high GI provide a surge of energy, so they're useful for people while they're exercising, but not so good for a sedentary lifestyle – or at least, not in large quantities.

Most green vegetables have a glycaemic index of 1 or less. Glucose has a glycaemic index of 100. Most other foods are somewhere in between. Animal products have a glycaemic index of zero because they have no impact on blood sugar level. What does all this mean for your weight? It means you can stop worrying about these foods and start eating. It's difficult to get fat eating low GI foods.

Most nuts and seeds have a GI of around 10 to 20. Most fruits have a GI between 30 and 60. Most beans and lentils have a GI between 20 and 40. These are really healthy, low GI foods, which you can eat without worrying about your weight.

Most grains have a GI between 60 and 70. Most potatoes have a GI between 65 (new) and 85 (baked). New potatoes are considered to be medium GI foods, and baked potatoes are high. Both have a bigger impact on blood sugar levels and energy than low GI foods and if you eat them in large quantities, you will probably start to gain weight. This is perfect for an anorexic who is ready to gain weight and get well, but not for a compulsive binge eater. Binge eaters who are looking to reach a healthier weight, would do well to eat more greens.

The glycaemic index is a useful way of understanding the effect of food on the body more broadly than just the calories consumed. Low GI foods tend to be nutritionally dense, good for your overall health and wellbeing. High GI foods aren't bad foods, but they do cause a surge in blood sugar levels, which means they have more potential to cause weight gain and obesity problems. They should be consumed in moderation, unless you're underweight. Medium GI foods sit nicely in the middle. They'll give you a healthy energy boost.

I find that understanding the GI of foods is helpful in making me realise that I can eat large portions of certain foods and not worry about surging blood sugar levels, diabetes or weight gain. But don't get paranoid about the glycaemic index of foods. If this knowledge helps you feel more able to eat a healthy meal, and alleviates your fear of all food, then becoming more familiar with the GI of foods might be helpful for you.

Counting calories

If you've had an eating disorder, you probably know the calories contained in everything off by heart. While many people do find counting calories detrimental to recovery, sometimes it can be helpful. When I made a real commitment to recovery, I found counting calories helpful, because, up to that stage, I hadn't given myself permission to eat any calories. I was frightened of all food, whether it contained one calorie or 500. Calories filled me with fear. However, by deciding that I would give myself permission to eat a certain number of calories per day, I allowed myself to eat. That was a big step forward. I gave myself permission to eat and to feel OK about eating. I didn't need to purge because I had permission. That helped me, but it won't be the right approach for everyone.

Some might think that hanging onto an obsession with calories is unhelpful. I get that, and it might be necessary to wean yourself off an obsession with calories, throw out the scales and just be brave and eat. But one way or another, you must give yourself permission to eat, managing the rising panic when you start to feel full, so you don't give in to the compulsion to purge.

As time passes and you start to feel more comfortable with what you're eating, you'll see that your weight doesn't shoot up. You'll feel able to introduce more foods, increase the quantities of what you're eating and, if you're still counting calories, eventually you'll feel comfortable enough to stop counting and eat more freely.

Getting away from calorie counting is something we all need to do eventually, but whether calorie counting is helpful or counterproductive for you, at this point in your journey, is something only you can tell.

Learning to eat again, without panicking can be a slow process, but it's very rewarding to eventually be able to go out for dinner with friends and not worry. Even if you do feel like you've eaten too much afterwards, just live with the anxiety, let the food go down and maintain a healthy lifestyle. Because choosing healthy foods and staying active are what will determine your weight in the long-term, not punishing diets, panic and social isolation.

What are healthy foods?

The healthiest foods to help you on the road to optimal nutrition and good health, are foods that have not been processed. This means they're in the same condition as they were when they came out of the ground, or off the plant or tree; fruits and vegetables, nuts, pulses and grains.

Animal products are also nutritionally dense, with oily fish being a front runner as a great source of omega 3. Organic foods are better still!

Industrial processing of foods for canning, making into ready meals and turning into cakes and pastries, reduces the nutrient content of the foods. That doesn't mean you shouldn't eat them. It just means that freshly made foods are healthier. For optimal nutrition, it's always better to make your foods from scratch, starting with raw natural ingredients. Many people feel better in themselves when they eat healthier foods and fewer packaged foods.

So make your interest in food about enjoying food for good health, rather than about restricting food in pursuit of some fake Western ideal of body image that makes you ill and, for most of us, is unachievable.

Nutritional supplements

Most doctors agree that nutritional supplements are unnecessary. But some nutritionists think that we should always take supplements because modern intensive farming methods have reduced the nutrient content of foods, so we need to top up. Scientific studies have conflicting views on this topic.

I would say that when you're recovering from ill-health, there's no harm in topping up with a supplement if you feel you want to. A decent supplement might give your body a helping hand.

If your weight is so low that you're dangerously thin, then shakes designed to increase body weight can be very helpful. You should be following medical advice if your condition is that bad – any food will help you, processed, liquidised, or otherwise.

One anorexic I came across, swore that zinc supplements corrected her distorted thinking and 'cured' her anorexia. The evidence for zinc supplementation in anorexia shows benefits, so it might be worthwhile if your doctor agrees. It's important not to overdose on any supplements. They can be helpful, but they can also be toxic in high quantities. Stick to the amount recommended on the jar, or advised by your health practitioner, and you should be fine.

Probiotics

Dr Campbell-McBride MD, author of *Gut and Psychology Syndrome*, takes the view that eating disorders are caused by unhealthy microbes in the gut, and she says the way to fix this is to go onto her special diet, which rebuilds the integrity of the gut wall and repopulates it with healthy bacteria. Key to her programme is the inclusion of probiotics, which are taken both as supplements and as fermented foods, including home-made sauerkraut, kefir, and probiotic yogurt.

Her programme cuts out grains and involves eating a lot of animal produce. Personally I think it's unwise for someone recovering from an eating disorder to engage in another very restrictive diet; however her suggestion to include probiotics in your diet makes sense as they may help reduce intestinal problems and discomfort.

Beyond that, I'd suggest that you do what feels right for you. There are many insightful books about nutrition and there's something to be gained from reading widely on the topic and making up your own mind about the best long-term approach for you. I'm not talking about diet books but about nutrition books, which are focused on good health, not on weight.

A healthy eating plan

So what does a healthy eating plan look like?

Well, it varies for each individual, depending on your existing weight, personal goals and any immediate threats to your health, but generally speaking, if your condition is not life-threatening, then the following healthy eating plan will give you a good starting point.

These are just ideas. If you have your own preferred foods, then add them to the list and create your own eating plan. If your preferred foods aren't so healthy, don't worry. The key is to start eating regularly, while consuming normal quantities of food. My focus on health is to make you realise that you can eat and not get fat. Obviously, eating donuts all the time will make you fat, so just use your common sense. Create your own eating plan and then give yourself permission to eat and enjoy it. Here are my suggestions:

Breakfast:

- A bowl of fruit with plain yogurt on top; or
- A bowl of muesli with milk; or
- Baked beans on wholemeal toast; or
- Egg on wholemeal toast.

Elevenses:

- a piece of fruit or a handful of nuts.

Lunch:

- A large salad with a wholemeal roll, hummus or another dressing, and cheese or meat; or
- Meat or fish, with vegetables; or
- A sandwich of your choice, plus an apple.

Mid-afternoon snack:

- a piece of fruit or a handful of nuts.

Dinner:

- A large vegetable dish, with cheese on top; or
- Meat and vegetables; or
- Oily fish with vegetables; or
- A pie of your choice with vegetables; or
- A slice of home-made nut roast with vegetables.

What you include in your meal plan isn't important. Most people recovering from eating disorders would probably prefer to choose healthy low calorie foods and that's fine. The important thing is to make sure you eat enough of them, so that you're not still starving, or inclined to binge (starvation dramatically increases your risk of a binge). So don't underestimate how much you can safely eat.

Ideally, you should consume plenty of vegetables – not just see them as a garnish. The government's five-a-day advice on fruit and vegetables is a *minimum* recommendation.

When you draw up your own meal plan, don't include foods that you know are likely to trigger a binge. Plan ahead and try to stick to your plan, so you don't overeat and regret it, or under-eat, leaving yourself hungry and prone to binge behaviours. You can adjust your meal plan once you get a feel for how well it's working for you.

If you do binge, don't panic. Just start again at the next meal time and stick to your plan. One binge won't ruin everything. Feel proud of yourself for getting a grip quickly and for not repeating your binge behaviour throughout the day. Resist the urge to vomit even if you feel uncomfortably full. Vomiting encourages overeating and will work against your efforts to stop binging and eat normally again. Keep the food down even if you feel nauseous. It's a necessary part of recovery.

When you're ready, introduce new foods, widen your choices, be less strict and let go of calories. Give yourself permission to eat out occasionally and relax, but don't let other people bully you into eating foods you don't want, which then make you panic and want to purge. Take your recovery at your own pace and you should be fine.

Learning to cook healthy meals

There are lots of recipes available online. Print out some of your favourite healthy recipes and cook them. Enjoy them. Relish the taste. Put some in the refrigerator or freeze it, to have the following day. One of the dangers of cooking is that you eat the lot when the recipe was designed to feed six. If you think bingeing is a risk, adjust the quantities in the recipe and cooking times. Only cook enough for your upcoming meal. Stay in control.

Learning to cook can help you appreciate healthy eating. If you don't like one of the ingredients, leave it out, or substitute. I frequently adapt recipes to make them healthier, using olive oil instead of butter, or leaving sugar out of the recipe because it's a savoury dish and I don't think sugar is necessary. Healthy sugar alternatives include dried fruit, juices or desiccated coconut. Adapt and be comfortable with what you're eating and cooking.

The main thing is that one way or another, you become comfortable eating again. You need to become at ease with the feelings food gives you. You need to learn to love your body enough to nurture it and feed it with healthy foods, rather than abuse it, starve it or overfeed it.

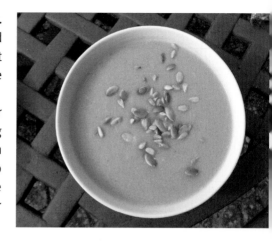

Love yourself and love your body. If it's the 'wrong' shape, so what!? There's more to life. In the section on recovery, we'll look at other interests, distractions and ways to get away from focusing all your attention on body image and weight, to gain a healthier outlook on life and on setting new healthy goals and finding happiness.

Chapter 12

Adjusting to Change

As you start to eat more normally again, you'll experience a period of adjustment, which is a natural part of the healing process. You may experience some digestive discomfort as your body adjusts to a regular eating pattern; you'll need to let go of the priorities that have kept you trapped in this way of life for so long. Embrace new priorities, like self-love, self-care and compassion for your body. You'll need to widen your outlook, find new interests and get a new perspective on the world. This will help to take your mind off body image and food. There is so much more to life than our culture's shallow ideal of how people should look! If your friends think there's nothing more to life than being thin, get new friends. You need to be surrounded by positive influences, not fashion victims who think the worth of any individual is determined by their appearance. There's more on meeting new people and finding new interests in the next few chapters.

Recovering from bulimia or binge eating disorder

If you're recovering from bulimia or binge eating disorder, it's probably early days and you're still worried about your weight. If you're feeling compelled to diet, remember that dieting hasn't worked in the past and is likely to increase the risk of a binge.

Stick to your meal plan with regular meal times. Your hunger signals are distorted, so eating regularly, rather than just when you're hungry, can help bring routine and normality back into your life. This also avoids grazing, losing track, panicking and then losing control.

So sit down to meals and savour the taste. Try to make it a pleasant experience. Focus on the moment, not the TV. Leave the table when you've finished eating to give the meal a distinct ending and reduce the temptation to eat more. Remember that it can take around twenty minutes before your body feels satisfied after a meal. If you feel bloated, don't panic. Your food will go down eventually and your hunger and satisfaction signals will normalise over the weeks and months ahead.

As your body adjusts, there will be some weight fluctuation (both ups and downs), so try not to become too anxious about it. Focus on getting well. You might find it easier if you wear loose fitting clothes, as tight clothes can make you feel more anxious about your weight and shape. Elasticated waists can be a godsend at this time. You're adjusting both physically and emotionally as you come to terms with accepting your body just the way it is.

Don't skip meals, because you risk making up for it by bingeing in the evening. Even if you're not hungry, stick to your regular routine. Feelings of hunger aren't reliable to a recovering bulimic, or someone with binge eating disorder.

It's common to relapse a few times. Hopefully you won't, but if your efforts to avoid bingeing have been unsuccessful and then you've purged, eat something small and nourishing to avoid it happening again. Put the episode behind you and consciously 'start again'.

If a specific cause can be identified for your stressful state before the binge, examine alternative ways of dealing with how it makes you feel the next time something similar happens. Discuss difficult feelings with a friend or counsellor, so that you have an outlet for those emotions, apart from your eating disorder. Allow yourself to cry and let it out. Therapy may help you get to the root of the problem. Explore alternative ways to comfort yourself when you're down.

If you've binged but haven't purged – DON'T! It won't make any difference to your weight in the context of a sensible diet. Just wait for it to go down and remember that tomorrow's a fresh new day.

Refusing to purge will naturally make your binges (and cravings) smaller and less frequent, so even a binge during a moment of weakness doesn't need to lead to the whole horrible cycle unfolding. On average, you have to eat 3500 calories to put on a single pound, so if there's evidence of weight gain the following morning, it doesn't mean it's permanent. Your body weight naturally fluctuates and some of that is water retention, which will pass. It's really not that easy to gain weight quickly, which is why your lifestyle and regular eating patterns matter more than what happens on one single day.

So resist the temptation to weigh yourself constantly. Changing water levels make daily readings inaccurate. Prospective weight loss will not show on the scales immediately and you may appear to have gained weight after a binge, but that effect won't last. If you weigh yourself weekly, at the same time, in the same clothes, you will get a much more realistic view of your true weight. Some people in recovery prefer to get rid of their scales altogether.

Stop trying to lose weight and concentrate on establishing a sensible eating routine whereby your weight remains fairly stable. When you eventually feel you have control over your eating, if you're not underweight and still want to lose a few pounds, you're in a better position to cut down a little, or eat more healthily. But it shouldn't be a diet. Diets don't work. It should be a lifestyle. Allow yourself treats, so you're not missing out, but decide in advance how much you will have – two chocolates for example. Give yourself permission to enjoy them and don't feel guilty.

While you're in recovery, you might feel more comfortable if there are no sweet foods in the house, because they're the most tempting binge foods. So shop when you're full so that biscuits and cakes are less enticing, but don't make yourself go without altogether. If your family are filling the cupboards with binge foods, ask them to help you by not buying them. A supportive family, willing to cooperate, is a great help. You can all get healthy together! Fill the house with fresh fruit and vegetables, rather than binge foods. If you fill up on green vegetables, you'll be less inclined to binge.

However, this is not an exercise in deprivation. Treat yourself from time to time, to a book, a cappuccino, a scone, or new clothes, so you don't feel that you're going without. If you're going out and feel vulnerable to binge, then leave your money at home, so you can't.

Don't prepare foods for other people while you're in recovery, as this puts more pressure on you to be in control around food.

If you become more vulnerable to bingeing in the afternoon, plan distracting activities as a preventative measure. Think about activities you enjoy that you can't do when you're eating. Take up interests, jobs, volunteering opportunities, or join clubs to make new friends. Friends will help to build up your confidence, so the more true friends you have, the better. You'll be out enjoying yourself rather than bored or bingeing. Try to focus on positive things.

Have a realistic view of yourself, accept your imperfections and remove 'should', 'ought', 'must' and 'if only' from your vocabulary. Finally, don't expect miracles right away. Be prepared for a slow and challenging recovery, but remember small steps in the right direction lead to a happier life, free of your eating disorder in the long run.

Recovering from anorexia

Perhaps you're recovering from anorexia but still feeling incredibly anxious about just about everything. Recognise that recovery is a long process, but it's worth it. When you feel bloated, it's not because you have eaten too much, but because you have eaten so little in the past, so your body is adjusting. That takes time, so be brave.

If you meet the definition of anorexia, you're severely underweight, so you should get personalised dietary advice from a dietician. It's very important not to lose weight as this could be life-threatening. You might find it helpful to draw up a list of your favourite foods and remember that 2000 calories is a normal healthy daily intake for a woman; 2500 for a man. Now give yourself permission to eat least three meals a day. Plan them with your dietician and stick rigidly to your plan. Set yourself specific meal times so that every aspect of your meal is pre-arranged and eat everything on your plan.

I found it helpful to start slowly, with foods and volumes I was comfortable with. Then I'd add another 100 calories to my plan. It was the next step in my recovery. I didn't gain weight from the extra 100 calories, but every small step was progress.

So give yourself permission to eat your meals and try not to panic. Over time, continue to add to your diet with help from your dietician. Introduce new foods and if you're struggling with the volume of food at one meal, try having five small meals per day instead of three. You won't feel as full as if the same food was consumed at three larger meals.

Look in the mirror and ask yourself what you *really* look like. Try hard to see what is actually there. Are your ribs sticking out? Are your limbs like matchsticks? It's not healthy and you're probably thinner than some of your idols. I used to admire Cindy Crawford – I thought she was beautiful. But Cindy Crawford was never as skinny as me!

If you're still convinced that you're fat, write down the physical evidence for this belief. Then write down the physical evidence for you NOT being fat. Look at the two lists rationally and don't disregard the evidence that you're *not* fat, because it's stronger. You should be able to see that. If you still think you're fat, but you're clinically underweight, discuss the evidence with a friend who you trust to be honest with you. They'll help you to see things the way they really are. Bones sticking out are not attractive and they show that you're skinny as a rake.

Your doctor should be able to refer you to a therapist or counsellor who's willing to listen to your problems in confidence. They may be able to put them in perspective and offer you constructive advice. Talk your weight concerns through with your therapist too.

Bear in mind that your anorexia has caused water retention in your body, which may add weight on the scales. When you start eating properly, your body will adjust to lose the excess water, so if you feel you're gaining weight, but the scales don't show it, this might just be the period of adjustment. If at some point, you do gain weight, don't panic – you're not fat. You're recovering, and this is a good thing. You'll feel good about this eventually, but it just takes time to adjust.

Get new interests, focus on the more important things in life, and try not to worry. Remember females, that you need to reach a weight whereby you menstruate, because if you don't, you are at risk of osteoporosis, which could leave you in a lot of pain and with limited mobility.

Look at your life and concentrate on finding something else to focus on: spiritual contentment, a hobby or a career move for example. What would you like on your gravestone? She was thin? Of course not. It doesn't matter. Try to find something to focus on that really *is* more important.

Chapter 13

Breaking Free from the Lure of Pro-ana Communities

One of the most alarming things about eating disorders since the dawn of the World Wide Web, are the pro-anorexia websites and communities that have emerged, encouraging young women, mostly, to pursue distorted ideas of beauty through extreme thinness. The websites glamorise eating disorders and tout anorexia as a lifestyle, not an illness. In 2013, the *Daily Telegraph* estimated that two-thirds of those affected by eating disorders in the UK have visited these sites at some time.

The websites tend to contain images of ultra-thin girls and phrases such as 'fade to nothing', 'make them regret calling you fat', and 'perfection takes time, so keep at it', to motivate young women trapped in the grips of an eating disorder. 'Thinspiration' inspires anorexic women to fight hunger and continue to starve themselves in pursuit of a higher goal: perfection.

How do people get sucked into pro-anorexia communities? These communities are designed to give people obsessed with being thin a sense of belonging, encouragement, drive and understanding. It can seem quite attractive and aspirational to someone who feels unhappy and misunderstood. Loneliness, isolation and not 'fitting in', are all risk factors for eating disorders. A sufferer may have felt alienated from society for a long time. So following pro-anorexia websites and forums can make them feel less alone, less isolated and may validate the way they feel about themselves, their weight, and their responses to problems. However, in order to break free from an eating disorder, an individual needs to find a supportive environment and healthy interests, elsewhere.

Fortunately, there are alternatives for the individual who needs this social reassurance and support, but is tired of being sick, hungry and trying to live up to an impossible ideal. A determined individual can show more strength by breaking free from their eating disorder, than by maintaining it. However, engaging with communities that glorify anorexia will undoubtedly hinder any attempt to get well.

For recovery to take place, the social gap needs to be filled. So initially, I'd suggest making a decision NOT to visit pro-anorexia sites and instead, start exploring the healthy alternatives to these social forums.

The eating disorders charity Beat has a number of support services available. They include supportive communities, both online and in localities around the UK. They have an adult helpline and a youth helpline. The understanding people at the other end of the phone are trained to provide support, information and let you know about treatment options. They might be able to direct you to services where practical help is available in your locality.

The charity also has online message boards and support groups. This enables you to find peer support in a non-judgemental setting, among people who understand what you're going through and who are on the same journey as you.

Furthermore, Beat has peer support groups running in local areas, so if there's one near you, you might benefit from meeting people locally who are struggling with the same issues as you. They aim to provide group support in a positive, therapeutic setting. This can be very helpful, and will help to reinforce your decision to break free from your eating disorder.

People engaged in pro-anorexic communities will feel better if they make a decision to re-engage with the real world and strive for a healthier lifestyle, which is not based on thinness, but instead, on good health, good relationships and happiness.

The truth is that the pro-anorexia websites can help to feed a condition that can be fatal, with up to 20 per cent of sufferers dying from complications relating to the disease. Even drinking too much water can kill you. Many participants don't realise they are building up a toxic cocktail of health problems, which can only be prevented, or minimised, by breaking free from their eating disorder, sooner rather than later.

Joining clubs and taking up new interests can be helpful too – generally people will be pleasant, chatty and engage you in their interests, if you introduce yourself and discuss the club's hobby.

It's always difficult trying to build friendships from scratch, but new interests will help you find purpose and a healthier focus, which will make it easier to break free from your eating disorder. Consider whether joining one of the following groups might help you:

- Your local youth club.
- Church - you might be surprised by the range of activities going on in some parish churches. Even if you find the Sunday services a bore, other activities that take place in the week can be part of a fulfilling social life.
- Photography club.
- Your local writing group or poetry society – writing can be very therapeutic and help you work through some of your emotional issues.
- Women's Institute – they're not all as old and boring as you might think.
- Countryside group.
- Volunteers society.
- The Ramblers.
- Local history club.

If you think they all sound boring, write down alternatives, but seriously, give some a chance. They're healthier past times than spending your evening starving and miserable, bingeing, or with your head down the loo.

They're also healthier than spending time looking at online images of emaciated women, which make you feel like you're not good enough. You are good enough. You always were. Get out into the real world and find people who appreciate you for the lovely person you are. It doesn't matter if they're young or old. You need positivity and kindness, not judgement and feelings of inadequacy.

Chapter 14

Recovery Strategies

Recovery from an eating disorder is a rocky road, full of pitfalls and uncertainties, but with every step, you're a little bit closer to breaking free from the disease that's taken over your life, probably for years.

One of the first things that will help your recovery is self-acceptance, just the way you are. Try to come to terms with your faults and imperfections and stop trying to improve your body. You need to learn to like yourself as an individual, accept your weaknesses

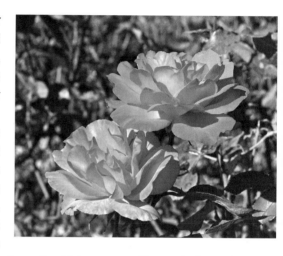

and, just as importantly, recognise your strengths. This way, you'll get a balanced view of yourself that isn't overwhelmed by a feeling of failure.

So, let's do an exercise. Write down your strengths – and don't say you don't have any. Everyone has strengths. What is your best subject at school, college, or your greatest strength at work? What do your friends like about you? Are you kind? Are you caring? Are you good with animals? If you really can't think of any strengths, or good personal attributes to be proud of, find a friend or therapist who can help you identify some, because getting some self-worth and self-esteem will help your recovery.

Then think about the things you like and value in other people. Most people are drawn to people who are happy, confident, generous and kind. People who are inspiring, creative or funny often have lots of friends. There is so much more to being a valued person in society than the size of your body. People aren't popular because they're thin. People admire confidence and wit, not a sad gaunt figure who's desperately unhappy.

So recognise that blind pursuit of thinness is not achieving the result you want. This will help you to break free. Happiness is not achieved by having a skinny figure, perfectly shaped eyebrows and a hairdo that takes two hours to get right every morning. Happiness is achieved by feeling comfortable within your own body, not trying to change it. Happiness is about spending time with people who make you feel good, doing things you enjoy, soaking up the sea air, playing games with friends.

If you can let go of this quest to be thin, then you'll be able to relax more easily and enjoy the pleasures that life has to offer. You'll slowly start to feel more confident and find new friends if you want to. You'll adjust to be the size your body wants to be and eventually, you'll feel you can trust your body and its hunger signals.

Focus on caring for your body, rather than trying to be thin. You will have more energy, your health will improve, you'll feel less emotional and you'll probably sleep better. Your appetite will normalise, your weight will stabilise, and you'll start to look more like the happy, confident person that you wanted to be all along.

It's a long journey and all of this isn't easy on your own, so visit your doctor and make the most of any help that is available. You've got nothing to lose by speaking to a counsellor or psychotherapist, if they're willing to refer you; you might have everything to gain. They could help you work through some of the underlying issues. Willpower and motivation in abundance are very helpful and important factors too.

Find a support group to help you break free

Support groups can be very valuable for people recovering from eating disorders, because they offer unconditional support and you'll meet other people in the same position as yourself, which makes you feel less like you're fighting this thing all on your own. They give you the opportunity to learn more about the risks associated with your eating disorder and about good nutrition and self-care.

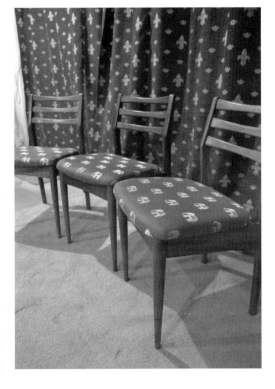

Groups enable you to express your experiences and concerns in a supportive environment, among people who share your anxieties, who are going through the same things and struggling with the same issues.

Some groups are run by NHS therapists at local clinics or hospitals, while others are run in the community by charities or individuals with a keen interest in helping people like yourself.

Different groups will have different approaches; some may be gender specific or focus on a specific eating disorder. Some groups focus on challenging negative thoughts to encourage more positive thinking, while others may work on addressing underlying issues such as self-esteem and self-expression. Some are focused on education, with a lecture format, a Q&A session, and a group discussion.

Groups are usually led by a qualified therapist, although there are some self-help groups led by unqualified group members, which are designed simply to offer companionship, support and sharing of information, as well as being an outlet for honest and open discussion and expression.

Groups can be comforting because you don't feel so alone or so misunderstood. The information disseminated in these groups can help drive your will and determination to recover and the other members provide valuable support. Eating disorder recovery is a long process and relapse is common, so it's good to have a support network where you can feel comfortable being honest about how it's going.

How do you find a suitable group? You can ask your doctor to refer you, or contact an eating disorders organisation, such as Beat, who have a network of local groups and other support services around the country.

Online forums for eating disorders

There are also a number of online forums for people with eating disorders.

ABC: Anorexia Bulimia Care is a UK organisation set up to help people recover from eating disorders. Look up their online forum, Health Unlocked, and join in their discussions. Some of the support on that site is excellent, and you'll immediately recognise other people going through the same things as you, and feel a sense of belonging. www.healthunlocked.com/anorexiabulimiacare

Beat is the UK's biggest eating disorders charity. They are there to inform, support and educate on the topic of eating disorders. Beat 'message boards' are there for people with eating disorders and their families and friends, to express their worries, seek support and ask questions about eating disorders, food, weight and shape. There are two separate message boards; one for adults and one for young people. www.b-eat.co.uk/support-services/message-boards

The Mental Health Forum is a friendly space for discussion, help and support with mental health issues; it has a specially designated eating disorders forum where people affected by eating disorders can express themselves, and their frustrations while looking for help and support among the community. This one doesn't require registration to view the comments, so you can see how it works, and get a feel for the atmosphere and feedback given, without signing up. www.mentalhealthforum.net/forum/forum32.html

Why Eat is a site designed to offer information, support and encouragement to individuals trying to recover from an eating disorder. The forums are separated into categories by eating disorder type, which might be useful for people with binge eating disorder, for example, looking to engage with other people who have that specific disorder. www.whyeat.net

The National Eating Disorders Association is a US organisation dedicated to supporting those trying to recover from eating disorders. Their online forums are separated into topics, including 'spouses of sufferers' and 'siblings', which might be useful for those groups of people looking for like-minded support. www.nationaleatingdisorders.org/forum

Organisations that offer support and advice
ABC: Anorexia Bulimia Care
www.anorexiabulimiacare.org.uk
Helpline: 03000 111213

Beat: Beating Eating Disorders
www.b-eat.co.uk
Helpline: 0345 634 1414
Youthline: 0345 634 7650

Overeaters Anonymous
www.oagb.org.uk
Helpline: 07000 784985

Finding a counsellor

Individuals with an eating disorder in the UK should be able to get some kind of help on the NHS. Cognitive behavioural therapy seems to be their favourite talking therapy, because it's thought to be effective and can be delivered in groups, which is an efficient use of resources. Access to eating disorder support groups may also be available through your doctor.

The NHS often offer group therapy first, only making one-to-one therapy available if it's considered to be necessary once group therapy has been completed. If at some stage NHS services dry up, or access becomes more difficult and you've run out of fight, then you might also want to look for counselling services locally to help you work through some of the underlying issues that have contributed to your eating disorder's development in the first place.

The charity 'Mind' offers counselling across the UK. It's subsidised, but the cost might seem a bit high to the low waged, especially as counselling is often ongoing and the costs accumulate. It's worth checking out what's available in your locality and weighing up your options. Some charitable organisations have been known to offer counselling sessions for as little as a fiver to the low waged and if you have special circumstances, then you might be eligible for free counselling.

Telephone counselling

The Samaritans

If access to counsellors is proving troublesome, there's always someone at the end of the phone when you call The Samaritans. They are there 24/7 to help anyone feeling in 'distress' or 'despair'. The old emphasis on them being there just to help the suicidal no longer applies, so don't feel that you're not bad enough to qualify for their help. If you need help, they're there to help. It doesn't matter whether you're depressed, struggling to cope, or worried about someone else. Tel. 116 123

NAPAC

NAPAC exists to support the adult survivors of childhood abuse. They have a telephone helpline, which is open on weekdays, and manned by counsellors specifically trained to help adults who suffered from childhood abuse. Tel. 0808 801 0331.

Childline

Children in need of support can call Childline, which is there to help youngsters who feel scared or vulnerable. They can offer advice on bullying, religious faith, your rights, self-harm and embarrassment. Tel. 0800 1111

New interests

For people with an eating disorder, the 24/7 obsession with food and weight is a real problem and it's particularly difficult to stop worrying about food and body image if you don't have other interests to occupy your mind. Somehow you need to get a new focus for your life; developing healthy new interests is a good place to start. Think about activities you might enjoy, that you're not engaged in regularly, and actively try to change that situation.

Also, look for activities that can help you to break free. For example, you can't binge if you're out on the tennis courts playing a game. There's no food. It's just you, the ball and your opponent. Pursue interests rather than indulging your eating disorder and the feeling may pass, or at least be delayed, perhaps reducing the frequency of your bad habits.

Keep busy. Go for a walk with friends or join a local walking group. Talk to new people and find out about their interests. Show interest in them even if you don't really care, because it might help you to make new friends and discover new interests. Who knows, you might even enjoy it!

Do some sport, join classes, try new things and accept invitations. If you feel you need to binge, take yourself somewhere that's totally distracting where you won't be able to binge – perhaps visit a friend, or offer to give a neighbour a hand with their gardening. Anything to quash that urge to binge and get you doing something constructive. Some people say the desire to binge is reduced by cleaning their teeth. Well, it's worth a try.

Coping with anxiety, challenging negativity and using distraction techniques

It's normal for someone with an eating disorder to be very anxious about food, eating and appearance, to feel guilty after eating and to be terribly anxious about the consequences of food consumed. It drives a feeling of panic, sometimes followed by fasting or purging. People with eating disorders are often anxious people generally, so it's worth knowing there are techniques that might help. They won't appeal to everyone, but you might find one or two of them helpful.

- When you start feeling anxious, stop what you're doing, sit down, close your eyes, and breathe slowly and steadily to help yourself relax. Focus on your breath, not the cause of the anxiety. Imagine a pleasant scene, or recall a happy memory and dwell on the good thoughts in detail (including sights, sounds and smells).
- Are you overwhelmed by negative thoughts? Challenge them! What is the evidence for and against your reasoning? Would someone else see it as such a problem? Try to replace it with a more constructive thought. Is there a healthy solution? If you can't change the situation, then look for a healthy way of distracting yourself from the difficult situation. Perhaps it's time for a walk in the countryside!
- Try to replace negative thoughts with positive ones, and reassure yourself with affirmations like: 'Things will get better soon. I'm as good as anyone else.' The theory of repeating positive affirmations every day is that even if you don't believe them to begin with, they will start to penetrate your subconscious and if you start to believe them, they are more likely to come true. So keep at it.
- Interrupt the rising anxiety by occupying your mind with something different. Count backwards from 100 in lots of three. Try to think of a different animal (or any broad subject) for each letter of the alphabet. Recall the words of a song, poem, or prayer. Describe the room, as if to a friend, in great detail. Some people find this helpful.

- Begin any activity that absorbs both your mind and your body:
  - Do a crossword or write a letter or email.
  - Get creative and make something you can be proud of.
  - Write a list of places you'd like to visit on holiday and research what you might see when you're there. Make plans.
  - Make preparations for your weekend, or a big event like Christmas.
  - Go online and enrol in a FutureLearn course that's just started. Participate in the course immediately to take your mind off your troubles. You'll meet new people and engage in positive activities while you're there. www.futurelearn.com

Avoid over-thinking

Some anxious people are prone to over-thinking. They think about everything that could possibly go wrong in a situation, which paralyses them from making decisions or taking risks – even tiny ones, like accepting an invitation out with friends. This can lead to misery and isolation and needs to be challenged. If you find yourself over-thinking, worrying about all the negatives that might happen if you take opportunities, try to focus on positives too, get a more balanced perspective and consider taking some risks. Sometimes it's necessary to take risks so that you can enjoy the fullness of life. I'm not talking about bungee jumping or potentially dangerous activity holidays, but just about

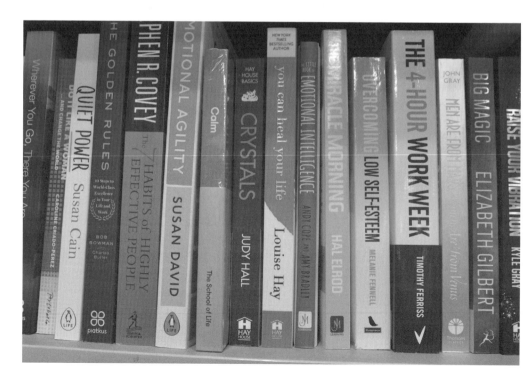

relaxing a little bit and trying new things; a new job, volunteering, new social activities and new hobbies.

Try not to over-think everything, because this can make you miserable. If you take opportunities and seek new experiences, you'll have a more fulfilling life and probably become happier and more confident. You might make friends and develop new skills. Don't worry that you might fail, you might not fit in, or you might not enjoy an activity. Try new things, and keep trying new things, until you find activities that are right for you.

Avoid negative influences

Are there some influences in your life that support your disordered eating behaviour? Do glossy magazines or the tabloid press make you feel like a failure because you don't meet their ideal? Swap fashion magazines or tabloid trash for a magazine focused on a hobby, like gardening, camping, crystals, or making things with beads. Perhaps avoid health and fitness magazines too, as these might add to your compulsion to achieve 'the ideal look'.

Do certain friends pressure you to look a certain way, make you feel inadequate, or criticise you constantly? Consider whether these relationships are healthy and in your best interests. Make new positive friendships, spend less time with negative influences and see if this improves your outlook on life and your self-esteem.

Try to dispose of the negative influences in your life where possible. You need supportive influences that make you feel good and worthwhile as a human being, not negative influences who put you down and make you feel like you don't match up.

It might help to do an exercise, writing down all the individuals influencing your life and whether they are positive or negative. Can the negative influences be replaced by more positive ones? Exploring your options here might seem a bit risky, but the outcome could provide a big boost to your confidence and self-esteem, which could change your life for the better.

Learn to love yourself

Learning to love and respect yourself, even when other people are unkind, helps to build the strength you need for recovery. Don't let people's thoughtlessness and unkind words get you down. Try to be strong in the face of adversity and if possible, avoid people who are persistently critical, unkind, or just plain nasty.

Focus on living with integrity and self-care. Surround yourself with supportive people and things that make you feel good. Write down some of the things you have to be grateful for, keep busy, and try to focus on the good things in your life. This approach will help you feel positive and more optimistic about the future. Then you can focus on new positive goals and ambitions for a brighter future.

Follow your dreams

I'm guessing that most people with an eating disorder abandoned their hopes and dreams long ago, amid feelings of utter hopelessness, despair and depression, accompanied by an inability to see any way to change things or envision a positive future. It was probably one of the things that drove you to an eating disorder in the first place.

Now that you're committed to recovery, it's time to rekindle some of your hopes and dreams. Perhaps some are still possible. What would you like to achieve now? Try to envisage a positive life in the future. What would you like to be doing? What subjects interest you? Would you like to go back to college? It doesn't matter if you've missed some years. It doesn't matter if you're middle aged and you want to try something new.

While many of my dreams and aspirations were thwarted and abandoned as a young girl, there was one dream I never entirely gave up on – my ambition to be a writer and to actually earn a living from my writing. I'll admit it took some considerable years after my recovery to find the confidence to become a full-time writer, but I've achieved it. And I work alone as a freelancer, so I don't have to put up with other people's unhelpful remarks, criticisms, dramas in the office, or bosses giving me a verbal whipping because I accidentally did something they didn't like. So I've achieved one of my dreams; perhaps you can too, with focus, hard work and dedication. Put all the effort you've put into weight loss into following a healthy dream instead, or into enjoying life. You might surprise yourself.

I read about a local woman who had always had a dream of acting, but life and other commitments got in the way. So, in her eighties, she decided to do something about it. She attended drama college, graduated, and then secured a role in a Hollywood movie. It was released a few years ago in cinemas across the UK. So it's never too late to follow some of your dreams.

When you get older, it's sometimes easier to follow your dreams than when you're young, because you're more in control of your life than when you were a child. Once you're an independent adult, it doesn't matter what other people think. Those with no ambition and no vision always ridicule those who set out to do great things with their lives. So surround yourself, as much as possible, with people who are kind and supportive; people who share your interests and attitudes. Make small steps and, if there's something you're not allowed to pursue right now, perhaps you can come back to it later. If there's something you're too old to pursue now, then perhaps there's another dream you can pursue, like I did. Some people will always disapprove but once you're independent, their view doesn't matter. You have willpower, integrity and determination. Not everything will work out, but at least you tried. You might have some modest successes along the way, even if you're not as successful as you'd hoped!

If you have aspirations to be a model, it might be worth knowing that statistically, you're more likely to die from anorexia than become a top model. So concentrate on reaching a healthy weight, so you're happy, you look healthy and then apply to be a catalogue model through a relevant agency, or see if your local photographic club can use your services. Start with modest ambitions and grow it from there. Don't starve yourself trying to get stick thin and famous. It really isn't worth dying for.

Perhaps you have no big dreams, except to be happy and free? That's great too. Visualise your life free from your eating disorder. What would you like to do when your thoughts aren't dominated by worries about food and weight? Travel? Have pets? Redecorate? Get a new job? Focus on healthy new goals and once you're able to visualise a better future for yourself, it might give you more strength and determination to break free.

Dealing with problems

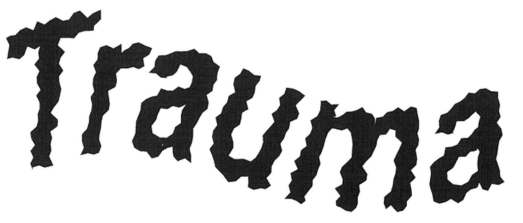

Eating disorders are often triggered by stress, trauma, or difficult experiences, and when things improve, or appropriate therapy is received, they release their intense hold on your life. If you ever feel you're at risk of slipping back into disordered eating, problem solving skills can help. One tried and tested approach to problem resolution is to write down your problems, then list all possible solutions, and the implications of those solutions. Getting it all down on paper can help you to assess your options, analyse them, and find the most acceptable solutions to you. Try it next time you're stressed because you don't know what to do. You might find putting all your options down on paper is helpful in clarifying the situation and the implications of any decisions you might make.

The importance of sleep

Getting a good night's sleep may be easier said than done, but sleeping well can make a big difference to your mood, your resilience and your ability to cope with life's unexpected challenges. Good sleep will also help you to beat your eating disorder. You're more likely to feel positive, keep your resolve and believe that the future looks brighter. So try to ensure you get enough sleep by avoiding caffeine in the evenings, going to bed at a sensible time and trying to create a serene atmosphere in your bedroom, which is conducive to sleep.

Overcoming a lazy bowel

Once you start eating sensibly again, if you're like me and you abused laxatives, you might end up very constipated. This is bad. When your eating is under control, you might find ground flaxseed, sprinkled on your breakfast, helpful in normalising your bowel movements. Flaxseed oil is an alternative to the ground seed. I relied on flaxseed for regular movements for years, before successfully retraining my bowel to work more normally. Flaxseed is an omega 3 oil, so it's healthy too. But do get your eating under control first because otherwise, there's a risk of it being ineffective. Ground flax will bulk out in your gut, so it should always be taken with fluids.

If you use flaxseed oil in large doses daily, as opposed to the ground seed, it can make your bowel even lazier. So do seek medical advice if you're needing to use the oil frequently, or in ever increasing doses.

Chapter 15

The Therapeutic Effects of Writing

When you're struggling with your feelings, and there's no-one to talk to, another way of expressing yourself is through writing. We've already looked at some forums where you can discuss your experiences with other people in the same boat, but writing in more detail about your own personal experiences can actually be quite healing.

Many people who have felt different or rejected have turned to writing as a form of therapy. It's a way of expressing yourself freely and without criticism. You learn to craft your feelings onto paper and sometimes this approach not only tells a great story, but it can be psychologically healing and even quite profound.

It's a way of analysing everything that's happened to you and understanding how it's shaped the person you've become. It can help you come to terms with it all and see how many seemingly insurmountable challenges you've overcome. Sharing your writing can help other people who are struggling with similar issues in their lives. Some people blog about their experiences, to reach out, get feedback and help others. Beware of online trolls though, who gain pleasure in upsetting people. Perhaps it's good to keep personal stuff anonymous, or within trusted forums.

There's a website called Cathartic, which exists to help people express themselves. It provides a form of release by allowing people to say the things that are perhaps unacceptable at home. The address is: www.cathartic.co. You might find it interesting. All users are completely anonymous, so if you register you'll get a user number and a password that you'll need to write down.

Writing is often adopted as a therapeutic tool by people who are prone to depression because it allows them to express themselves in a non-threatening way. Therapeutic writing comes straight from the heart and it challenges the status quo in our society, which frankly, sometimes needs to be challenged.

There is a lot of research which shows that writing can be therapeutic and beneficial to people suffering from trauma. It can even be beneficial to those suffering from everyday stresses, to help them work through their day-to-day challenges.

Therapeutic writing offers a way of getting your emotions out into the open, providing a release mechanism for suppressed feelings, which may have been bottled up for years. It may help reveal solutions to problems, or identify new ways of coping with difficult feelings.

Even the editing process is said to be therapeutic, because you can hone and perfect the words until you're completely comfortable with the message portrayed – that's something you can't do in talk therapy when you might express something badly and later wish you'd expressed it differently ... or perhaps not said it at all. Honing your writing can bring out the raw truth in a situation and help you to analyse your feelings and understand why situations make you feel so bad. It can also help to put things in perspective, by enabling you to focus on the challenges you're facing and take a balanced look at your life.

With writing therapy, you can work through emotions, without fear of judgment or of igniting an inflammatory reaction from those who may not see things in quite the same way. There's no need to share your writing, but obviously you can if you want to. Some people find that burning their writing is a symbolic way of putting the past behind them and saying, 'now it's gone'.

Richard Pelzer, the brother of David, the most abused child in America, said that writing his book was therapeutic. It's a way of addressing feelings of mistreatment or abandonment and working through what happened. It can be very beneficial and can help you see different perspectives, which may provide a greater sense of understanding too. In times of economic hardship and government cuts, where access to traditional therapies is at an all-time premium, writing is free and accessible.

In 2005, researchers Baikie and Wilhelm, published a paper entitled 'Emotional and physical health benefits of expressive writing' in the medical journal, *Advances in Psychiatric Treatment*. Their work looked at the numerous studies published on the topic of writing as therapy and found that for most people, writing about your painful experiences for just 15-20 minutes a day, for three to five days, can help to improve your emotional wellbeing.

However, it's also possible that the therapeutic writing experience may be upsetting in the short term, so if you find this, you should reconsider whether it's the right approach for you. It doesn't help everyone; one study showed that certain groups of traumatised individuals had an adverse effect to the writing process, so individual response is an important consideration. Some people suggest that writing memoirs should be done in close collaboration with a therapist who is there as a sounding board whenever you need one!

Baikie and Wilhelm added that, despite bringing up some upsetting memories, the therapeutic writing experience provides a release that is beneficial to the writer in the longer term. So the long-term benefits of therapeutic writing include lower stress levels, improved immunity, lower blood pressure, better physical health and a sense of wellbeing. It may also reduce the risk of depression and post-traumatic avoidance behaviour. In addition, the research shows that the process may increase a person's chance of finding employment, reduce their absenteeism at work, improve their memory, improve their grades at school and improve their performance in sports. It's really quite remarkable how effective therapeutic writing can be.

According to Smyth in 1998, a drug that could achieve the same benefits as writing therapy would be regarded as a 'major medical advance'.

Do check out the Cathartic website at www.cathartic.co and start expressing yourself in a small way if you want to. Or keep a journal, just for yourself, if you think it might help.

Chapter 16

How Should Parents and Families Respond?

Accept that recovery is a very long and slow process, and it will take time for the eating disordered person to fight their demons and make good their recovery.

Don't nag them. My mum nagged while I was in recovery and her continual whine, as it came across, was of no help at all. Being told that bingeing is stupid and then asked why you continue to do it, only confirms every bulimic's opinion of themselves; stupid and out of control. Don't nag them to stop – it isn't that simple – and don't nag them to eat more. Instead, make them feel welcome at the dinner table, regardless of whether they eat or not and let them know that their company is valued.

If you're helping your anorexic daughter or son with a re-feeding programme, agreed with a therapist, try to ensure that the food is something they'll enjoy – this way their ordeal is no more horrible than necessary.

When you feel irate and want them to 'snap out of it' remember that they know their behaviour is stupid, ridiculous, senseless and all the other things that you're likely to yell. Confirmations of their hopelessness are of no benefit to either of you.

Instead, be there to listen when they need someone to talk to and try to understand without judgement or criticism. If you've read this book and don't understand why these things happen by the time you've got this far, then you probably never will, so don't persist in making the sufferer feel like an idiot. Make them feel they can be open with you and trust your confidentiality. Then be honest, but not brutal, about your concerns for them and let them know you're there to support them every step of the way.

If they react badly, understand that they're just confused and hurting inside. Be completely accepting of them, just the way they are. Total acceptance from you will help them to accept themselves.

Lots of tempting foods left all around the house are the most awful thing to cope with for a bulimic trying to overcome their cravings, a binge eater, or an anorexic who's terrified of food. Put chocolates and cakes away – in fact, put all the food away. It's best if you don't buy lots of high calorie sweet foods either, because a bulimic might be terrified to venture downstairs, for fear of being overwhelmed by a compulsion to consume the whole lot and then purge. Try to stock healthy foods that they feel they can cope with, and don't fill the house with sweet foods that they'll struggle with.

Don't give the sufferer larger or smaller portions unless they have asked you to. Differential treatment makes them feel unnecessarily self-conscious. Try to avoid confrontations over food.

Do find out what help is available in your area and encourage them to take any opportunities for help. Whether it's through your local doctor, mental health services team, or the eating disorders charity Beat, there are many people and organisations, who might be able to offer some kind of support and assistance.

Don't say to the sufferer that they look better when they have put on weight because they may well panic, believing that if their weight gain is noticeable, they must be getting fat. By all means compliment them on their appearance, but NOT their increase in weight.

If they go off the rails, lie to you or do things they shouldn't, try to be consistently supportive. People do funny things during times of extreme stress. They just need unconditional love and support to get through it.

Beat has adult carers support groups around the country, which you might find helpful if you're finding it tough and could do with a support network of your own.

Chapter 17

Jennai Cox

Jennai Cox used to suffer with anorexia nervosa, starving herself in pursuit of an unattainable physical ideal. The turning point came when she realised how much she was upsetting the people who loved her. It gave her the strength to break free.

'Mirrors tell lies,' explained Jennai. 'They reflected not what I expected, but what I wanted to see. Me – fat'.

'I was never really overweight, so when and why my obsession started was something of a mystery.' Jennai didn't consider that she had a problem, even though she was anorexic for two years.

'I told myself that I was not sick, strange or different, as all the concerned looks kept telling me. I never once admitted to anyone that I was on a diet. It gave them the reassurance they wanted and the protection I needed. Occasionally, brave friends would make a cautious remark about my having lost weight, but instead of alerting me to my condition, this would fill me with the happiness and sense of achievement so lacking in other areas of my life. It just made me more determined to go on.'

Jennai became an expert at fending off comments about her appearance. 'It was just a symptom,' she explained. 'What I dreaded and avoided was being confronted with the cause – the truth. Even so, something in the pit of my hollow stomach was crying out for someone to forget about the weight loss and ask about me.'

Her experiences growing up were typical of someone who develops with anxieties about their weight: 'As far back as I can remember, my mother was always on a diet. She once made me hold bags of flour equal to the amount of weight she lost. My father never showed me the affection and attention a daughter needs. During ten years of ballet concerts, violin recitals and school plays, I do not remember seeing his face more than twice in the audience. Being the eldest of four girls, I was the first to experience puberty, which at bath time made me the subject of much teasing.'

'At 15 I was very aware of myself, physically and mentally. I did not like it, and neither, I thought, did anyone else. If anyone had ever expressed alarm about anything except my outward appearance I might have been able to reveal the intense unhappiness, dissatisfaction, even disgust I felt with my life and myself.

'At heart, I was no more enjoying experiencing my condition than others were witnessing it. What I saw as perfecting myself on the outside was compensation for the inadequacy I felt inside. To a degree, the feeling of losing weight filled that gap. But my defensive and light-hearted treatment of any concern that was voiced, masked the agony underpinning my condition and kept probing questions at bay.

'My anorexia was an addiction. Not so much to thinness as to the feeling of self-control. But the price of that power was high. I can still remember the nausea of going for days without so much as a water biscuit. The constant fatigue and rattiness, of even running out of the energy to pretend I was feeling fine.

'Getting away with not eating was easy. Like many people I never had breakfast. More often than not, I skipped school dinners, and at home I always said I was doing homework and would eat later. I never did.

'I alienated everyone, dearest friends and closest family. I withdrew, protected by barriers of deceit and cynicism, and lived a life of self-inflicted secrecy. It took a great deal of effort, a fair share of pain and many tears to unburden the guilt of knowing I was responsible for the damage I had done, and could have done, to my life and the lives of those around me. Any genuine desire to recover meant forcing myself to recognise the selfish nature of anorexia.'

As Jennai became more aware of how concerned her family and friends were about her condition, she started to realise things needed to change. She didn't want to keep hurting other people.

'The intense worry of my family and friends, which deep down I knew was simply waiting to erupt, had been there all the time. I chose to ignore it. My father would give me periodic lectures about how thin I looked, the fact that I dragged my feet as though I never had any energy and always looked miserable. "Your sisters keep asking me what is wrong," he would say. "Can't you tell me?"'

When her mother made me an appointment to see her GP, Jennai grudgingly went along. 'Having anticipated the sort of check-up the doctor would give me, I went along swaddled in layers of clothing and carrying bags of money in the hope that when I was

weighed, the scales would tip a little way past reality. I was referred to a psychologist who, after questioning me about my childhood, still could not tell me what was wrong, or why. I assured her I would start eating more and never went back. During all these ordeals, whether with parents or doctors, the word anorexia was never mentioned.'

Jennai never confessed to being at fault, but realising the pain she was causing caused her to reflect on her life. 'I was wrong to think that

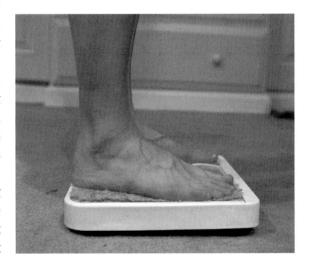

what I was doing was not affecting anyone but myself. I hurt people terribly – people I loved – and realising this was the turning point.

'Witnessing the effects outside myself changed my attitude inside. I cannot remember when it happened, but the unhappiness and fear for my life that had, until then, simmered just beneath the surface, suddenly boiled over. My mother was crying hysterically, unable to sleep through worry for me. My sisters were all deeply upset and had even read a book about anorexia to try to understand what had happened to me. Behind the silence and concern were love and care I had never realised existed – at least not for me.

'To say this was the turning point does not mean I could immediately start eating normally again. Both mind and body had to get used to the reformed attitude, and reconciling the two was not easy, but once the mind is made up, the hardest part of the battle is won. The rest is perseverance.'

Jennai fully recovered from her eating disorder and went on to become a successful writer, and owner of a drama school. She never really understood her anorexia fully, saying, 'I can recall and explain my horror at the sight of a meal, the guilt of swallowing a mouthful of potato, but as to why it started or how it could have been prevented, I am none the wiser. Anorexia is an illness, but it is self-inflicted. Nobody can force a person to starve themselves when food is in ample supply. But even when an ulterior motive exists, something still has to tip the balance. If self-dissatisfaction is the root cause, factors contributing to it must be looked at. There is no doubt in my mind that the bombardment of images of model-thin perfection can adversely affect vulnerable adolescent girls and boys. To those already feeling unhappy or insecure, anorexia seems the easiest route to outside perfection, especially when a kind of self-satisfaction comes with it.

'I can now happily eat a three-course meal without a twinge of remorse. For me that is an accomplishment. But I may not have been here to tell the tale had it not been for the tremendous support, encouragement and love I received from friends and family who, although ignorant of my condition, cared enough to do something. To them, I will always be grateful.

'I might still be strong willed, but with sufficient memories and a few photographs to remind me of that ghost like existence, I do not have the will to go through it again. In any case, mirrors are a good deal kinder to me now. So am I.'

CREDIT: All quotes in this chapter were written by Jennai Cox.

Chapter 18

Sarah's Battle with Anorexia Nervosa

I met Sarah when she was 16 years old. It was the mid-1990s and she was a year behind her former classmates at school because she'd spent so much time in hospital. This is her story.

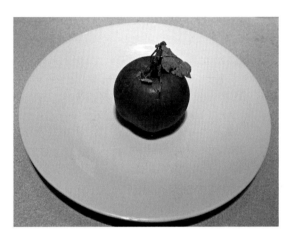

At the age of 5, the carefree childhood that Sarah knew ended swiftly with a twisted perversion that she didn't understand. She went to spend a week with her grandparents and it was the first occasion of many to come, when she was sexually abused and raped by her grandfather.

'My grandfather changed from the old man who bounced me around on his knee, to a total bastard who abused me. I hated him,' she said. 'At the age of 5, I vowed that I was going to kill him. I didn't understand what he was doing to me, but I hated it. He said he was doing it because he loved me. He said everybody did it and said if I told anyone, they'd laugh at me, because it was normal. In the back of my mind, I knew that it wasn't right, but I didn't know it was wrong. I didn't know what it was. I went home at the end of the week and everything felt different. I really wanted to tell mum because it hurt and I was bleeding all the time, but I couldn't because I thought my mum would laugh and say, "This is part of life."'

Then her parents started arguing incessantly, so she threw herself into her school work. When she was 6 or 7, the family moved to London. She lost contact with friends and was bullied at her new school. 'Everyone used to call me a snob and brain box,' she said. 'I hated it. I didn't have any friends.'

Then one day, she was sitting on her teacher's lap, begrudgingly reading a story. Her teacher kept hugging her and Sarah hated being touched, thanks to her grandfather. So she grabbed the teacher's thumb and yanked it hard, bending it right back and breaking it. This led to her first experience with a psychiatrist. She sat on the floor playing with the surgery's toys, while her parents spoke to him.

Back at school, the teachers and children alike were bemused by Sarah's behaviour. She ran away frequently and refused to wear school uniform. At other times, she was a model pupil. She threw herself into her school work to take her mind off her problems and, inevitably, this brought pleasing results for her otherwise bewildered teachers.

Sarah's grandfather continued to sexually abuse her, but now that the distance between them had widened, she didn't see him very often. This was a relief, but provided little comfort when they did visit.

When she was 10, the family moved again, but Sarah had trouble settling in, feeling lonely and isolated. 'The other kids thought I was a really hard city girl,' she complained, 'and after living in London for three years, the countryside was unbelievably boring.'

Sarah was almost 11 years old when she first started to feel guilty about eating food. She started to think that life would improve if she was thinner, but she snacked secretly between meals. As feelings of guilt around food developed, her grandfather's abuse became increasingly intense.

The following September, when the new school year began, things started looking up. She became more popular at school and visits to her grandparents became something of a rarity. But family life came tumbling down at home and her parents decided to separate. It was an emotionally-fuelled, spur of the moment decision which was short lived. They got back together again a few weeks later. Then split again. It was to become something of a habit. They had another trial reunion but the stormy relationship continued.

'Things got really, really bad at home. There was constant arguing and my mum beat my dad up and threw things at him. My brother was very depressed.'

Sarah lived in a part of the country that still had grammar schools and secondary schools, so at the age of 11, she took the 12+ examination and failed. All her friends passed and she was gutted. Off she went that September, to her new secondary school, where she worked obsessively, and was then bullied for working hard and being a bore.

'My goal was to get to the grammar school, because that was where I felt I belonged,' she explained, but the bullying intensified and became more personal. 'People started saying, "You're really fat and you've got big boobs",' said Sarah. 'That made me very conscious of my body and what I was eating. Then we did a project on healthy eating, which made me even more aware of my diet. I started throwing my lunch away.'

The problems at home continued. Her life became focused on food, because she could control it and this helped her cope with everything else. Her hard work paid off and after a year at secondary school, she was transferred to the grammar school at the age of 13.

Meanwhile, her parents kept walking out on each other and then returning home to make up. One day, Sarah spotted her father embracing another woman. Not wanting to cause more fireworks at home, she kept the secret to herself, but her eating habits deteriorated rapidly. She reached a stage where she almost stopped eating altogether and started exercising excessively.

'I was so obsessed with school work, exercise and food, that it became my life. The rest of the world didn't matter. The more I got into it, the more lonely I became and the more

I wanted to break out, but I couldn't – because I was so caught up in it all. My whole goal was to lose more weight – get thinner and thinner. I'd say to myself, 'You can cope. The thinner you get, the better you'll be. If only you lose another stone, then you'll be happy.' But I'd lose another stone, still be unhappy and then I'd want to lose more.'

She was becoming irritable and felt furious with anyone who interrupted her exercising. She felt guilty if she ate and tried to hide the extent of her exercising, but if she missed the bus to go swimming, she'd stomp home, slam all the doors and refuse to speak to anyone, except to bite their heads off. Then she'd go to her room and exercise. Her rapid and extreme weight loss became alarming.

That winter, the cold turned Sarah's skin a deathly white, almost blue, but she still refused to acknowledge her problem. Her friends at school tried to get her to see Matron but she wouldn't, still insisting that there was nothing wrong with her. She shivered all the time and wore four pairs of gloves to try and keep out the cold. She survived the winter on very little food, drank sugar-free Ribena and lemon tea, but would still not acknowledge her problem.

Then her mum walked out. Sarah was left with her dad and shortly, he and her mum were arguing about who should keep her. Neither of them wanted her. 'My dad was saying,'"I don't want you to live with me" and mum was yelling, "Well I don't want her to live with me!"

'Then one night, after mum had moved back in again, she was terribly depressed about everything. She locked herself in her room and I knew that she had a bottle of pills in there. I didn't know what to do. I kept knocking on the door saying, "Mum, let me in," but she wouldn't. She was crying and I honestly thought she was going to take this overdose, so I rang one of her friends who's a psychiatrist and said, "Come over, Mum's going to kill herself!" She came over and mum went to live with her for a while and took my little sister with her.'

Then a friend of Sarah's brother moved in because he was being beaten by his parents. He introduced her to recreational drugs. By the time she went to Germany on a school exchange trip, she was a low weight, needy and in a very bad place emotionally. An unwanted sexual experience in Germany brought back all the horrible feelings about her grandad. She was only 13.

By now in a state of complete turmoil, Sarah was using her body to hide her pain. She returned to Britain feeling violated, regretful, and broken. 'I couldn't face telling anyone,' she explained. 'I just find it really embarrassing and I don't want to dig up the dirt. I'd rather forget it because I know that if I had to go to court and testify, I'd get really upset. I don't want my parents to know about it either.'

When the school term ended and the summer holidays began, Sarah took an overdose. At six-and-a-half stone, she was referred to a psychiatric clinic, where she tried to kill herself by taking more overdoses and slashing her wrists.

Perhaps unusually for an anorexic, Sarah wasn't concerned specifically about weight at the time. She had an obsessive desire to be thinner, but was so unconcerned about her actual weight, that she never knew how heavy she was. Her actual weight only began to concern her when she noticed that it seemed to be of concern to the doctors.

'My weight didn't really bother me until doctors started weighing me. Then I convinced myself that five stone – yes, that's a really normal weight. That's a FINE weight. I was completely convinced.'

As the school year began again that September, she was 14 and still losing weight. 'I didn't stop eating because I thought I was fat. That was just an excuse for it. Really, it was just my way of coping. I felt that if I didn't eat, then I'd be stronger somehow and a better person – that I could face the world. I suppose it was a way out, an escape route. I knew that if I didn't want to concentrate on all the really awful things in my life, I could just concentrate on food.

'I'd think, "Right, I've eaten 100 calories today, I can eat 50 tomorrow, and 25 the next." I'd calculate every calorie. I'd wrap myself up in the world of exercise and food. I had a total obsession with food and my whole body was just craving food. I used to spend hours looking at cookery books and cooking elaborate meals for my family, which I never ate. I planned diets for my friends, so they'd have exactly the right balance of nutrients, but I'd be sitting there with a can of diet coke. My friends became really worried.'

Rightly so, because Sarah's weight had dropped to four-and-a-half stone since her referral to the clinic. Their methods obviously weren't helping. She was admitted to a specialist unit.

'When I was four and a half stone, logically, my brain was saying, "Don't be stupid, you don't need to lose weight at four and a half stone. I mean you're what? Five foot five? You're not fat at four and a half stone! It's impossible." But it wasn't what I believed inside. I believed I needed to be thinner.'

Sarah basically just believed that she could never be thin enough to cope with all the misery in her life. She was also terrified of fully developing a woman's body because she thought it would attract more sexual abuse.

'No-one's going to want to do anything to me because I'll be so ugly,' she recalled her thoughts of the time. 'That was one of the main reasons why I struggled against putting on weight. I was scared of what would happen. I kept up the pretence and when size 8 clothes were much too big, but I'd still say, "Urgh, I'm so fat!" I felt that I had to keep up this act.'

At the age of fourteen, shortly after starting the new school year, Sarah was admitted to a specialist eating disorder hospital as an inpatient. She was put on bed rest and had to stay in bed, all day, every day, unless she needed to use the bathroom. Even those trips were supervised, which she found utterly humiliating.

She wasn't allowed to make or receive phone calls, keep personal belongings, have letters or visitors, because she had been put on 'reward punishment', a system whereby the patient gets rewards as she puts on weight. Under 'reward punishment', belongings and nice things are withheld until they gain weight. As they gain weight, they are given rewards accordingly. It usually provides the patient with a strong incentive to eat. However, for Sarah, 'reward punishment' was not incentive enough. She refused to eat anything. It didn't help that the food was far from appetising.

'The vegetarian meal was potato pie and then you'd have potatoes with it! You'd have this really gross stuff to drink, like a syrup. It's really gloopy and it's got two and a half calories per millilitre. We used to have to drink three hundred millilitres of it. It's just SO gross!'

So she sat in her hospital room, containing nothing but her bed, hating her existence and wanting to die. A week later, she'd lost another four pounds and downy hair had grown all over her body. Downy hair is the body's response to chronic starvation; the body grows extra hair to keep it warm.

The hair on her head was coming out in large clumps when she brushed it. Her nails all broke and her feet were covered in horrid sores that wouldn't heal. She used to cut herself a lot, hack away at her body and slash her wrists, so she had scars and cuts all over her. They wouldn't heal either, because she wasn't getting any nutrition. The staff didn't know what to do with her, so she was moved to another hospital where she was tube fed.

'When I was first tube fed, I didn't realise what was happening. They grabbed me and shoved a tube up my nose. It was horrible so I kept pulling it out and they said, "If you do that once more, I'll tie your hands up," so I thought I'd better behave.

'After that, I didn't have any choice about what I ate. Even if it was something I really hated, I still had to eat it. It was awful because you had forty minutes to eat and if you hadn't eaten it by the end of that forty minutes, you had to sit at the table for another hour and a half. No-one was allowed to talk to you. You just had to sit there and if after that time, you still hadn't eaten it, they'd make you sit there for the rest of the day. All your meals would pile up, so you'd have your breakfast, your mid-morning snack, your lunch, and so on! If by the end of the day you still hadn't eaten all your food, they'd tube feed you.'

Sarah was forced to consume 3500 calories per day, which caused many sleepless nights because she felt so bloated. She'd been surviving on an apple a day until then, so it was a shock to her system.

'It was horrible because the first week or so, when I wasn't eating, I used to sit at the table all day. There'd be all this food in front of me and I used to get up from the table and run off, down the corridor. Someone would bring me back and sit me back down at the table again.'

When bed rest ended, and supervision relaxed, Sarah continued to exercise at every opportunity. She also made herself sick as often as possible after tube feeding. The anorexics were supervised for forty minutes after meals, but the staff didn't seem to realise that it was still possible to bring the food back up after this time. 'So we used to run down to the toilets and all the anorexics would be in there, being sick.'

Sarah's potassium levels, blood pressure and heart rate all became dangerously low, so she was put under stricter observation and treated for her physical problems.

Two months later, she returned to the previous hospital, where they fed her 4000 calories per day until she reached five stone. She was deeply depressed. Anti-depressants, tranquillisers, and sedatives, did little to help and it wasn't long before she began running away and overdosing, so she was put under constant observation again.

'It drove me absolutely insane!' she said. But she wasn't in any condition to look after herself. When she was discharged to go home for three weeks, she promptly stopped eating completely. Her weight plummeted, so her parents sent her back to hospital.

She spent a total of nine months at the hospital and reached a high of seven stone. She was discharged as an outpatient and her weight plummeted, but she refused to return. 'The whole regime was like a prison,' she explained. 'No one cared about what I felt, what had happened to me and why I was like that. It was just, "You're a low weight, you don't know your own mind. You've got to put on weight." That was the one thing I couldn't do. No-one would help me. If someone had actually bothered to say, "Well, do you want to talk about it? Why do you think this has happened? Why don't you want to develop a woman's figure?" then maybe I would have been able to accept the weight that I'd put on, but no one did. It was just, "You're going to kill yourself. Let's put you under constant observation and lock you up in a room. Oh, you've been naughty, we've got to give you an injection to calm you down. You've got to stay here, you've got to eat this, you've got to do that." It was so disciplinary, I couldn't take it. I felt like a prisoner because I wasn't allowed anything. I couldn't even go to the toilet by myself. No one really helped me. It was a complete nightmare.'

She ran away to London and slept rough for a while, before finding a hostel and settling in there. It wasn't long before the police found her and took her back home. She was still a minor. She was taken to the local psychiatric unit for a forty-eight-hour assessment.

'My friends came to visit and we went out walking, shopping and swimming – it wasn't like being in hospital at all! They did a blood test, asked me to complete two questionnaires, and then said I should be an inpatient.' It wasn't what she wanted to hear. She stormed off and started self-harming again, shouting, 'I'm dead already! I don't see why they don't just bloody well shoot me!' So she was readmitted to the psychiatric unit, but discharged herself the following day.

When her weight dropped to four-and-a-half stone, she was sectioned for six months. Still only 15 years old, she was their youngest patient. Back on bed rest, she was only allowed out of her room for half an hour a day to watch television, except to use the bathroom. She felt angry, trapped and constrained. 'The hospital had never had anyone with anorexia, never had anyone my age and didn't know what they were doing with me,' she said bitterly.

A diet of 5,000 calories per day was scheduled, much to Sarah's horror and disbelief. In an attempt to enforce this, she was given food supplement shakes every half hour, but refused to drink them, complaining that 5,000 calories was completely unrealistic when she hadn't been eating for months.

Then, to her surprise, people actually started talking to her. She saw a psychologist, and drew up a meal plan with a dietician. She was happy to start eating again on the terms they'd agreed together. She felt up-beat and positive about her experiences and made a positive effort to consume her diet. But she still wasn't allowed out of her room for more than half an hour per day, so she took overdoses and then stopped eating.

She went up and down in weight, seeing various specialists and being tube fed. Her sleep was badly disturbed by nightmares and at such a low weight, her body was screaming for food. But she still longed to be thinner. She was dosed up on sleeping pills, felt like a zombie and was unable to co-ordinate herself properly until about noon.

Then one night, still weighing just four-and-a-half stone, she ran away, took 100 paracetamol, cut her wrists, and then laid down to die. Police found her lying beside a lake and took her back to the hospital. She spent two weeks in intensive care before being sent to a private clinic for specialist treatment. It was a totally different environment.

'It was a lovely hospital and I had a really nice room,' said Sarah. 'I had a lovely doctor and it was so much better. I ate all my meals in my room with a nurse. This was so much better than having to eat with other people, which made me anxious. I was in an eating disorder ward, so there were lots of other people my age with the same problem.

'When I first arrived I was really depressed, so the doctor put me on loads of drugs and tranquillisers. I was doped out of my mind half the time, so I didn't know what I was doing. I was fed up with that, so I misbehaved and ended up in an observation room, with windows all the way round. The bed was screwed down, the TV was screwed down and I couldn't open the window properly because it would only open about an inch. It was like a padded cell. If I was really lucky, I was allowed out in the enclosed garden.

'A lot of the other people were also in observation rooms, in their pyjamas, so we used to go out in the garden and dance around. The nurse was worried that we'd escape, so we'd pretend to climb the wall and they'd come running after us!'

Sarah had regular psychotherapy sessions and was seen by a cognitive therapist. At long last, someone was showing concern, not just for her weight, but for the way she felt inside. They discussed the feelings that she'd had towards food and her body, and she found it very helpful.

'If I had a thought, say, *I am fat*. I'd then have to write down the evidence to support the thought; my thighs are big, for example. Then I'd write the evidence for not being fat. Like, I'm in hospital with treatment for anorexia and I'm three stone, or whatever! Then I'd have to write a rational comment on the two evidences. That approach really helped me, because it made me look at both points of view, weigh them up and see which one made sense. It made me start to think about who I really was. Then we started to deal with all this stuff about my grandad and the rapes, being bullied at school and being really unpopular.

'When I told my doctor about the sexual abuse, it was a big deal. It was something I'd never thought I could tell a man, but he was very easy to talk to and he was ever so good about it. He was an amazing doctor and I saw him every day which was great. There were lots of group therapy sessions too, including assertiveness, and three eating disorder groups a week. My counsellor was an ex-anorexic and bulimic. She had recovered for ten years, so it was really good to have someone who actually understood. The staff were wonderful.

'There weren't any stupid rules like having to be on bed rest and having to lie with your legs straight. We could go out in the garden, and go for walks. We used to go to the pub and restaurants. It was really good.

'We had art therapy where we explored our feelings through art. You'd have a theme, like having to draw all the good and bad things that had happened over the past year and then analyse it. We did cookery once a week to try and get used to food. We hid the butter and threw it out. Then we fried things, but wouldn't put any fat in the frying pan!'

At the clinic, they laid on tempting meals that included a starter, a main course and a dessert, so it wasn't necessary to keep having supplements throughout the day. Sarah was expected to eat everything that she was given, but she didn't mind because the food was delicious and they were granted as much time as they liked to eat it all.

As Sarah's eating habits improved, she was allowed to go down to the main dining room, decide what meals she would like, and serve herself. Eventually she reached her target weight of nine stone, but all this extra weight was alien to her and she felt terribly fat. Now she was able to eat without any difficulties or feelings of guilt, but she didn't feel she could cope with the weight gain.

When she left the hospital after six months of treatment, she immediately began losing weight. But under the threat of having to return to hospital, she forced herself to eat and stabilised at eight stone so everyone was happy. She returned to school, was pleased to see her friends and her confidence crept back. But she'd missed so much of the work while she was in hospital, that she was moved down a year, meaning she was practically a stranger to her classmates.

At home, she was now living with her mother and younger sister. Her father had left home a year earlier to live with his girlfriend, and her brother had gone to university. Although family dynamics were difficult, she said, 'I get on with my dad a bit better now that he's left.'

She continued to run every morning, swim four evenings a week, cycle and walk a lot. She still worried about food, and when asked whether or not she thinks she will ever be able to eat normally, Sarah replied, 'I don't know. I'd really like to be able to do that, but I don't think I ever will until ... When I started at the clinic, I needed longer to really start to come to terms with all the things that had happened to me. There's so much pain inside and I get so lonely and depressed. I really need someone professional to talk to. The problem is, I can't go back now because our insurance has run out. I'd love to go back and carry on where I left off.'

However, arrangements were made for Sarah to return to the specialist clinic that helped her so much, and she eventually made a full recovery.

Chapter 19

My Struggle with Bulimia Nervosa

I t was my first day at school. I was 4 years old, anxious and I didn't want to be there. Within days, bullies had locked onto my insecurities and were thumping me, excluding me, and saying unkind words. I avoided the bullies as best I could, but as years passed, things got worse, not better.

I didn't understand why no-one liked me. I was a quiet kid, very self-conscious. I was worried, always worried about something, and trying very hard to fit in. I was kicked, thumped – generally battered and bruised by the bullies, who worked in gangs so I was outnumbered. I didn't fight back.

I received a lot of abuse for not keeping up with the changing fashions and begged mum for the latest accessories – to no avail – but while I desperately wanted to conform, I did wonder whether owning the right 'stuff' would have made any difference. They hated me and it seemed nothing I could do would change that. When I walked home on my own, the bullies followed, blocking my path, pushing me into bushes or walls, and yelling abuse.

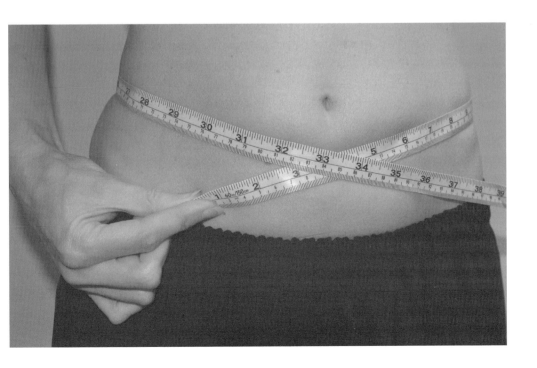

The teachers thought I was being awkward when I sat alone for fear of getting battered shins beneath the table and when the teacher left the room, I was driven into a corner by girls kicking me while the class cheered them on. Reporting was futile. The school weren't interested.

I developed a woman's body two years before everyone else. It was the subject of much mockery and teasing. They tried to pull my swim suit down in the pool and one of the teachers wanted me to parade topless at the class assembly! Mum let me take the day off.

Constantly on the edge of tears, I was called 'waterworks' at home by my parents, who would say 'Oh, for goodness' sake stop crying!' which just made me feel worse. I tried really hard not to let it out, bottling up painful feelings.

During those early years, my dad became my worst critic. He laid into me daily, criticising, ridiculing and belittling me. And because he was my dad, his words hurt deeply and crushed my self-esteem. I was constantly trying to change myself to please everyone around me, but nothing I could do was ever good enough.

Dad's criticism got so bad that mum phoned his brother, wanting to know how to make him stop. Dad's criticism was destroying me. She'd tried to challenge him, but their screaming rows, while I cowered in my bedroom, seemed to have little effect. My uncle said that's how my dad behaves. You can't stop him. I was only a little kid. He was a grown man in his forties.

After dishing out endless criticism, dad would scold me for crying. Both parents would 'give me something to cry about' – usually 'a good hiding'. Compassion seemed to be in short supply. I just didn't feel loved.

I wanted to prove to people that I wasn't the worthless failure they all thought I was. I was ambitious. I watched Olympic gymnasts on TV and dreamed of being there one day, but when a friend asked me to attend her gymnastics class, I wasn't allowed. I dreamed of being a ballet dancer when I grew up and begged mum to let me attend lessons, but she said no. So while friends went to various classes, I sat at home, unhappy, trying to convince myself that ballet was bad for your feet, so I didn't really want to do it anyway. And that success didn't happen to people like me, so I was stupid to entertain such ideas.

When I raised contentious issues, Mum said, 'I'm not interested and I don't care.' I wondered why my parents had bothered to have kids as they didn't seem to like them very much.

I thought about suicide a lot, but I was terrified of death and frightened of going to hell. I was also afraid of ending up disabled, instead of dead, so suicide was very risky, and I didn't do risk – I was far too cowardly.

The non-stop bullying meant it was hard to concentrate on my academic work. So I failed the 12+ exam, and went to the local secondary school. The bullies were there too. They were confident, fashionable and popular. They made new friends and their gang grew in size. A couple of my old friends joined their new gang. I was stunned.

They constantly criticised my appearance, calling me 'ugly' and 'pizza face'. My spots were quite bad, so I tried a sugar-free diet, various cleansers, and medicines. Nothing helped.

When I was 14, one of the bullies dragged me down the stairs by my hair, kicked me hard until I fell reeling to the floor, then continued to kick me while her mates cheered. I curled up, trying to cover my face from her flying feet. I wasn't a violent person at all. I just wanted to be left alone.

At home, my sisters were taking ballet classes and doing gymnastics. We heard all about their fantastic lessons over tea. I begged mum to let me join the same classes, but she said no. These were my sisters" 'things'. It was heart-breaking. She refused to discuss it any further.

I was allowed to join the church youth group. It was cliquey and I didn't fit in, but I enjoyed the outings and I'd trawl through photographs of the places we'd been, because it helped me feel better.

By the age of 15, I was desperate for a break from the school bullies. So I put on a big act, fooled around and became a disruptive class member. I wanted to show everyone that I had bags of confidence, that I was not as timid and pathetic as they all thought. Surprisingly perhaps, it helped. My level of social acceptance increased. Pretending to be confident, actually gave me a bit of real confidence. I felt slightly more resilient. But not much.

As part of this new act of confidence, I tried to block out painful emotions and pretend I didn't care. I was genuinely sick of the unkind, judgemental, bigoted attitudes in a society that seemed to determine people's worth by whether or not they were confident, charismatic, fashionable, or had all the latest gadgets. I'd been bending over backwards trying to fit in and please other people, but always failed. Nothing I could ever do was good enough. I started to feel it was our culture that was at fault, not me, so I stopped trying so hard to fit in. I felt better for it, but the merciless bullying continued. I wasn't *that* tough.

A new girl at school invited me to go to a rock disco ten miles away. So I went along, met loads of new people and felt completely exhilarated by the chilled out atmosphere, amazing welcome and total acceptance of me, just the way I was. None of them had any preconceived ideas about me and they were all so friendly. There wasn't an unkind word or a criticism from anyone. They just wanted me to join in the fun. It was fantastic. I went to the rock nights every week, was popular and I felt at home there. I'd never experienced unconditional acceptance like this before.

Perhaps it was predictable then, that Dad wouldn't approve of my new friends. While rock nights made me happy in a way I'd never experienced before, Dad took one look at the people who'd accepted me into their peer group and branded them all lazy, unemployed, layabouts ... because they had long hair, rock T-shirts, leather jackets and (God forbid!) a motorbike if they could afford one. Most of them were in sixth form and there was a nurse, a carer, a couple of lads who worked in Sainsbury's, an engineer and an accountant among them, but my dad wouldn't listen.

In September 1989, aged 15, I got my first boyfriend. Our relationship started well, but he frequently said he thought I was fat and his criticisms made me self-conscious. He finished with me three months later, Christmas Eve in fact, on the grounds that he'd met someone else.

So that new year, at ten stone, I began dieting. I saw weight loss as something positive I could achieve. I thought it would make me more attractive – perhaps make me more lovable.

I began refusing biscuits after lunch and puddings after dinner. I stopped buying chocolate bars and lost about a pound every fortnight. A month of deprivation later, the unnoticeable weight loss was very disappointing. I needed to diet harder, so I only allowed myself very small meals and lost weight at a reasonable pace. But instead of focusing on school work, I was starving myself and worrying about my weight.

The church youth group closed, so rock nights were my only social activity. The evenings gave me such a buzz that I looked forward to them all week. They were so successful that the landlord decided to hold them twice a week. I was over the moon ... until Dad picked me up one night (I usually got the bus), took one look at my friends, and banned me from going back. Ever.

So for the next few weeks, while my friends went to the rock nights, I sat in my bedroom on my own, desperately unhappy, trying to figure out how I could get away from home. I was convinced that my life was over.

It was a few weeks later when Mum was downstairs screaming at dad: 'What's she supposed to do? Spend her life in her bedroom? The church youth group's closed. She has no-where else to go!' It worked. For once it my life, sanity prevailed. I was allowed to go back to the rock nights. Until Dad set a ridiculous curfew, which would have forced me to leave at 8.30, half an hour after the rock disco began. Another blazing row ensued. I won, but I hated the fighting. I just wanted to be allowed to be happy. I wasn't coming back late. I always got the last bus home at 10.40.

I was still dieting when I noticed cellulite on my thighs. I'd bunked off PE at school; I hated it because I was bullied on the sports field, my shins were deliberately bashed black and blue with hockey sticks and no-one wanted me on their team anyway. I was always the last one standing when the teams were picked and the team who got me groaned.

I loved doing individual sports at school; athletics or gymnastics for example, but we only did them once in a blue moon. Usually it was team sports, and I was bullied. So, I avoided the lessons and when my thighs turned to jelly, I just thought I needed to eat less.

I was reading an article about the eating habits of a top model and the number of calories she consumed every day. Part of it referred to slimming, suggesting an intake of 1200 calories per day. I decided to try this and was surprised by the amount I was able to eat. I wasn't so drained of energy, but progress was slow, so I reduced my calorie allowance and eventually reached my target of nine stone. But my tummy still stuck out and I had cellulite on my thighs, so I dieted harder, lived on as little as possible and quickly became fed up and hungry.

Lack of sleep was just part of my life. Repetitive thoughts, trauma and anxiety about bullying had kept me awake long before hunger added to the problem. Chronic period pains and heavy bleeding kept me awake too and I suspect I was anaemic, like my mum. I'd watch the clock: 2am, 3am, 4am. Then I was woken at 7am by my sister's stereo. She slept like a log and didn't care. Surviving on two or three hours' sleep became normal. I felt exhausted and totally beaten.

I still thought that being thin enough would eventually make me more acceptable to the people who hated me, and perhaps to Dad, whose bitter criticism, constant ridicule and put downs had continued daily for the past decade.

At 16, I'd left school and was looking for a job. I'd been saving pennies from my Saturday jobs since I was 14 years old, and desperately wanted to move out because I needed the freedom to be myself, without criticism. But the recession of the 1990s had just kicked in and jobs weren't easy to find. I was trapped. Two months later, I was bored, depressed and had a huge collection of rejection letters. Rather than offering guidance and support, Dad was making my life miserable. Now I came into the 'unemployed layabout' category.

I don't remember a time when I haven't felt like a big disappointment to my dad, but during the summer of 1990, it was made particularly clear that I was wholly unacceptable to him. I applied for every job in the local newspaper, spent all my Saturday pay on stamps sending out applications and walked to the local shops and businesses, asking for work. But by September, I still hadn't found work; my confidence was at rock bottom.

English was my best subject at school, so I had aspirations to work in journalism, but the local paper wouldn't have me, there were no relevant courses at the local college and Dad said I was stupid to want to be a journalist anyway. Desperate, and out of options, I enrolled on a full-time engineering course on the day the course began; engineering jobs paid well and there were skills shortages, so I should be able to get a job at the end of it. It was a bad decision. I couldn't understand the maths and failed the first exams.

It was early October 1990 when things went from bad to worse. I had the house to myself one evening. I'd been on diets all year and was starving. I binged.

Afterwards I felt over-full and had terrifying visions of my weight rocketing overnight. My stomach had shrunk. I hadn't eaten that much, but I was panicking. I made myself sick. Just the once, I thought, but it became a habit.

After that, I was losing weight at an astonishing rate and felt a great sense of achievement. But I was also disgusted with myself and ashamed of my methods. I purged daily, then several times daily. It was the only way I could satisfy my appetite without putting on weight.

The weight fell off, but my appetite became insatiable and I had these horrible cravings. All day, every day, the only thing I wanted to do was eat. I was obsessed with food and terrified of it.

My appearance suffered dreadfully and within a few weeks of being sick, my eyes looked grey and burst blood vessels around my eyelids caused a horrible puffy redness. I blamed the inflammation on the harsh winds, which admittedly, were making them worse. The skin became very dry, cracked and flaky. It was very painful. I wanted to stop vomiting but was caught in an addictive cycle, hungry and needing food, but not feeling able to control it. I was still desperate to be thin, so I could be loved. When my weight dropped to seven and a half stone, I felt like I was really making progress, but at a horrible price.

I got a job in a stationery store but needed medical treatment for my inflamed eyes. My new employer objected to me taking time off to attend a doctor's appointment. After three weeks, they sacked me.

I tried to fight my bulimia, but every day was a battle. First I was driven by hunger; then I was driven by sheer terror. I binged and purged up to three times a day. They weren't all big binges though. Some weren't really binges at all. I was just terrified of eating anything and felt completely out of control.

Two months, hundreds of applications, and tens of interviews later, I was offered part-time work in the kitchens of a local hospital. It was the worst job ever for someone in my position, but I was desperate for work and applied for just about everything. Bingeing became easy surrounded by food at work.

I tried desperately not to give in to the cravings and often drank endlessly to avoid eating. I sometimes purged at work. Nurses used the hospital toilets and I remember fearing that one of them might realise what I was doing in the next cubicle. I was panicking again, terrified of food. I desperately wanted to stop and felt thoroughly ashamed of myself, but I couldn't bring myself to tell anyone.

My problem became a physical rejection as well as an emotional one. I was so used to having an empty stomach, that I physically felt nauseated if there was any food present in my stomach. My weight dropped to seven stone.

I finally found two months' work at a dentist's; away from food, which was a godsend. Keeping busy all day – in a job that didn't involve food – kept me in control. I could eat a little bit and not binge or purge. But when the work ended, I needed support so I didn't go downhill again.

I opened up to a few of my friends, hoping that removing the secrecy would help me on the road to recovery. It didn't help much. In fact, I think it turned some people off. They didn't understand. The people who really needed to know were my parents. They knew I was bingeing – the missing food was a source of irritation – but I think they assumed that I'd been fasting to make up for it. I was always 'on a diet'.

In April 1991, I went to a concert, got crushed, and collapsed. My head was swimming and I felt drunk – except I hadn't had a drink. My vision started to fade and all I could see was millions of little black specks dancing before my eyes. Then everything went black. It was weird! I couldn't see a thing yet my eyes were open and I was still fully conscious. It was scary; as I sat on the floor, the giddiness slowly subsided. After a few minutes my vision gradually returned. But the following day, I thought I'd broken my ribs. The pain was excruciating. I made an appointment with the doctor and went along to the surgery that afternoon. On inspection she told me that it was just severe bruising. Then she asked me when I had last made myself sick. I was taken aback, felt embarrassed and denied everything. I wasn't ready to admit to having an eating disorder.

I now weighed just over six stone. Technically, that made me anorexic, but I thought I had bulimia. I looked at myself in the mirror and I knew I looked awful. My ribs stuck out, my chest was practically non-existent, my cheeks were thin, almost fleshless. My limbs were like match sticks and the bones stuck out painfully. Despite my unnaturally thin body, I was amazed that even at this weight, there was still some cellulite on the remainder of my skinny thighs. It took me this long to realise that it was due to lack of exercise and nothing more. Ten minutes of daily exercise got rid of the cellulite in weeks and I knew I had to stop this destructive eating before I reached a stage beyond recovery. It was a turning point.

But change was going to be hard. My mind was totally absorbed by my eating disorder. It numbed the pain, loneliness, and hopelessness I was feeling. It stopped my periods and stopped the debilitating menstrual cramps that lasted weeks. It took away my sex drive, so I didn't feel so needy. But I was desperately unhappy and knew it wasn't a solution. I wanted my parents to notice and nurture me, but being thin didn't help. My eating disorder was suppressing my pain, but it was causing so many other problems, I wanted to stop. I wished I could, but I felt trapped in a terrifying cycle and unable to just stop.

In June 1991, I joined a scheme called 'Youth Training'. I wasn't keen because the scheme seemed exploitative to me, paying just 85p an hour for me to work full-time, doing sales administration for a commercial company. At that time, even the low waged typically earnt £3.50 an hour in employment. But I was now 17 years old, had been out of school for a year and was desperate. I'd had a few dead-end jobs, nothing new was on the horizon and I felt like I had no other option. I got day release to college from September onwards; being back in a full-time occupation and away from food, did help me get my eating under control.

I made a new start. I took small packed lunches, ate at lunchtime, consequently felt sick most of the afternoon (because food made me nauseous) and then did my best to keep sensible control over my eating when I returned home. I cut down the number of times I purged to about three times a week. To my horror, my eyes got worse. They were so painful, but eventually the appearance of my eyes did start to improve too. I gradually put on weight until I reached seven stone.

Just before my eighteenth birthday, the rock nights ended suddenly. My social life dried up. I didn't feel I could afford to go to the new pub where people were meeting. It was miles away, public transport was expensive and I suspected I couldn't get away with ordering tap water from the bar, which is what my life had been reduced to, on such low wages, while trying to save money for my escape from the hellish environment at home.

I tried to salvage a social life closer to home, but it wasn't very successful and I became lonely, demoralised, resentful about working full-time for less than £1 an hour, with a four-hour daily commute! So I started applying for jobs again.

Six months later, in June 1992, I was offered a six-month contract working in local authority payroll. I took it, but I hated the job, made some bad mistakes, lost all confidence and was no better off financially after I'd paid for the travel to work, paid my parents and been stung for basic rate tax (which was never refunded). Everything I did to try and change my circumstances seemed futile. I ended up back on 'Youth Training', typing and filing, while finishing my course in the evenings.

I battled with my eating disorder, having good days and bad days, eventually deciding that self-humiliation was the only way that I was going to be able to put an end to this awful addiction. So one evening when I was alone with Mum and Dad, I finally told them my terrible secret. They hadn't suspected a thing and seemed more bewildered than shocked. I felt so stupid. That was why it helped a lot. I made myself tell Mum every time I made myself sick and every time, I felt totally stupid and thoroughly humiliated.

So, committed to total honesty, the thought of having to admit my actions provided an effective deterrent, which enabled me to really start facing up to my problem and fighting it head on. I was no longer pretending it didn't exist. It took incredible determination and I felt physically awful for about a month. I felt sick all the time, but I knew I had to keep the food down. Because of this, I didn't eat very much and remained seven stone.

At seven stone, I was happy with my weight. It took me another year of ups and downs to gain complete control over my eating and every day was a battle. I tried to ignore the cravings and if I did give in, I'd live with the consequences. I refused to purge or fast. Yes, I'd be really uncomfortable for the rest of the day, have difficulty sleeping and feel awful in the morning. But I was determined to get well.

After a year, now at seven-and-a-half stone, I found I could consume about 1600 calories per day and stay absolutely stable. It ensured that while I wasn't gaining weight, I wasn't too frightened to eat either. There were ups and down, but it helped me a lot. It gave me permission to eat, without being afraid. Even then, for a year or so, I wouldn't touch any food that wasn't savoury.

A relapse came when I allowed myself the occasional small pudding or piece of chocolate and lost control. The cravings got worse, my resistance weakened and I tried desperately, to regain control. More ups and downs ensued, followed by sleepless nights; sometimes in longing, sometimes in discomfort, but importantly, I wasn't sick.

When I finished my youth training scheme in June 1993, I couldn't get away fast enough. I resented feeling exploited for two years in dead-end jobs and gutted that five months before my twentieth birthday, I was still getting less than £1 an hour. I didn't feel valued at all. On the upside, I'd got good grades on the course, which made me think that perhaps I had a future.

Unfortunately, however, employers didn't see the value in my grades or the so-called 'work experience'. I was really disappointed and after a horrid binge, I made myself sick for the first time in over a year. My feelings of self-revulsion and stripped dignity came flooding back, as did my eye problems – red and jelly-like by the following morning. I vowed that I'd never be sick again.

I was depressed, ate too much and rapidly put on a stone. I felt terrible. I hated myself. But I wouldn't allow myself to be sick.

I urgently wanted something to counteract my bingeing and turned to laxatives. When my stomach emptied out, it was an overwhelming relief and I thought I'd be able to start again. I had every intention of eating properly and exercising strict control over my diet again, but it didn't last.

I went up and down like a yo-yo and the laxatives ceased to have any effect. I eventually asked my doctor for help and got a place on a self-help group.

Two days later, I started part-time work at a new department store. I was motivated, keen to start again and I ate reasonably sensibly. I was bingeing less, keeping my food down and coming to terms with the fact that I would probably be a bit heavier than I wanted if I was to continue eating fairly 'normally'.

In November 1993, the self-help group began. We shared our experiences, supported one another, and received helpful advice and information. Socially, things were improving too. I joined a church and made a few new acquaintances. I felt valued.

Another turning point was when Mum received a letter from a friend of hers who had become osteoporotic after the menopause. Her friend was confined to bed all the time. She could hardly move and could do very little for herself. It made me look at myself – I hadn't had a period for four years because of the weight loss. I didn't want osteoporosis too! Was thinness really worth the agony? At about that same time, I saw a Christian Aid leaflet and looking at the starving people in Africa, I realised how stupid my obsession really was.

That was when I decided that if necessary, I'd be fat. I realised that even obesity would not be as bad as the utter hell of bulimia. Besides, I needed to put on some weight in order to begin menstruating and hopefully, avoid osteoporosis.

By 1994 I was eight-and-a-half stone and my eating had improved dramatically. I still binged occasionally, but they were only little binges and I was never sick. The cravings were nearly all gone and the enormous burden had lifted. If I did over-eat, I was finally able to not worry. I was fully prepared to be fat if that's what it took to wave goodbye to bulimia. The greatest thing was, I'd hardly put on any weight and I seemed to stabilise at eight-and-a-half stone.

Over the next few years I did fully recover and the desire to binge disappeared. I realised that there were much more important things in life and focussed on them. I did a psychology degree, hoping to help people like me. That didn't work out, so I retrained in marketing, qualified in nutrition, and eventually became a full-time writer. For those with the determination to recover, the future is bright!

Chapter 20

Hope for a Brighter Future

Breaking free from an eating disorder is a liberating experience. It enables you to channel your thoughts, time and energy into things that make you happy, bringing a sense of joy, fulfilment, and wellbeing.

While eating disorders may serve a purpose for a while, they don't provide any solutions. They can actually keep you trapped in a spiral of despair. So it's worth grabbing your future with both hands and finding the willpower and determination to break free.

You are a wonderful person, with strengths, hopes and dreams. Even simple dreams, like happiness, are realistic for everyone. So focus on healthy goals, take any help that's available, and be proactive in your recovery. If you fall down, start again. Life is full of ups and downs and recovery from an eating disorder is no different.

You can't change the past, but you can build a better future. Painful experiences from the past don't have to determine your future. Try to think positive thoughts and surround yourself with people who make you feel good, if you can. Be kind to yourself. Do things you enjoy. Take one small step at a time. Focus on recovery and consider how you might be able to fulfil some of your healthy, positive ambitions. Write down things to be thankful for, and keep a record of the progress you make during recovery. This can be helpful on a bad day, to help you see how far you've come.

Don't let other people's negativity get you down. You're worth more than that. Love yourself. Focus on positives. Learn new things; learning opens new doors and can be a life-enhancing experience. Take control of your life. Stay strong, and say goodbye to your eating disorder. Most importantly, I hope you can find lasting happiness.

Good luck. x
Louise

Follow me on Twitter @LouiseVTaylor

Acknowledgements

Thank you to the people who've helped me with this book by sharing their stories. I hope that by being open about our own struggles, we can help others to break free from their eating disorders and live happy, fulfilling lives.

A Selection of Books That You Might Find Helpful

AKHTAR, Mirian, *Positive Psychology for Overcoming Depression*, Watkins Publishing, 2012.

ARON, Elaine N., *The Highly Sensitive Person: How to Survive and Thrive When the World Overwhelms You*, Thorsons, 1999.

FENNELL, Melanie, *Overcoming Low Self-Esteem*, Robinson, 2009.

HOLFORD, Patrick, *The Optimum Nutrition Bible: The Book You Have To Read If Your Care About Your Health*, Piatkus, 2004.

JEFFERS, Susan, *Feel The Fear And Do It Anyway: How to Turn Your Fear and Indecision into Confidence and Action*, Vermillion, 2007.

JONES, Peter, *How to do Everything and be Happy*, HarperCollins, 2013.

SANFORD, Linda T., *Strong at the Broken Places: Overcoming the Trauma of Childhood Abuse*, Virago, 1991.

WALKER, Pete, *Complex PTSD: From Surviving to Thriving: A Guide and Map For Recovering From Childhood Trauma*, Creatspace, 2013.

WILSON, Pippa, *Letting Go of Ed: A Guide to Recovering from Your Eating Disorder* O Books, 2011.

Index

Abuse, 2, 29–30, 40–2, 45, 86, 121
  child, 42, 99, 106, 113–14, 116, 119
  emotional or psychological, 42
  laxative, 4, 9–10, 16, 23–4, 72, 104
  sexual, 42, 55
  substance, 40, 62
Anorexia, 2, 8–10, 14–6, 18
  biological causes of, 33–8
  conventional treatments for, 54–5, 57, 60–1
  culture and, 28, 30–2
  environmental factors and, 43, 45–8
  health risks of, 22–6
  Jennai's story, 112–17
  my story, 5–6, 127
  new treatments for, 64–6
  nutrition for, 76–7, 79, 81, 83
  pro-ana communities, 91–2
  recovering from, 89–90, 96–7, 102, 108
  Sarah's battle with, 113–20

Binge eating disorder, 11–12
  biological causes, 36
  conventional treatments for, 55, 61
  health risks of, 23
  new Treatments for, 64–5
  recovery from, 87–8, 97
Bulimia, 2–3, 8, 10–12, 14, 16, 18, 108
  biological causes, 34–8
  conventional treatments for, 55
  culture and, 30
  environmental factors and, 44, 46, 48
  health risks of, 22–4
  my story 5–7, 121, 126–9
  nutrition for, 83
  recovering from, 87–9, 96–7
Body dysmorphic disorder, 48, 66–7

Children, 30–1
  Childline, 98
  effects on, 31
  eating disorders among, 1, 30
  experiences as, 15, 40–4
  therapy for, 56
Constipation, 4, 9–10, 24, 72–3, 104

Depression, 4, 6, 8, 10–12, 14, 26
  complimentary therapies and, 70
  conventional treatments and, 53, 60–2
  elderly people with, 32
  environmental factors and, 40, 43, 45, 47–50
  new treatments and, 65, 67
  nutrition and, 76, 79
  recovery and, 102, 105–6

Elderly, 30–2

Family, 45, 50
  dynamics, 40
  genetics and traits, 33
  Jennai's story, 111–12
  Sarah's story, 113–14, 116, 120
  support, 89, 108–9
  therapy, 56–8, 60

Great starvation experiment, 20–1
Gut and psychology syndrome, 50, 83

Health risks and complications, 22–6
  bowel complications, 4, 8, 24, 72–3, 104
  candida/fungal infections 4, 25, 50
  cardiovascular, 4, 22–6, 32, 117
  death, 4, 22, 26, 32, 34, 76
  eye Damage, 3–4, 22, 25, 29, 126–7, 129
  malnutrition, 4, 22, 25, 26, 30, 56
  osteoporosis, 3, 24–5, 90, 129
  overweight/obesity, 11, 17, 21–3, 26, 50, 81
  renal complications, 23
  shock, 25
  stomach problems, 4, 10, 12, 16, 23, 26, 78–9
  tooth decay, 4, 24
Highly sensitive person, 49

Lazy bowel syndrome, 4, 24, 72, 104

Men, 1, 14, 20–1, 25, 44–6
  culture, 28, 31–2
  food and sugar addiction, 37
Middle aged, 1, 30–1

Post traumatic stress disorder or PTSD, 41, 49, 53, 55, 70

Pro-ana, 91–3
Purging disorder, 12–13

Stress, 2, 11, 20, 29, 33, 35, 103, 109
   Abuse and neglect, 42
   Change, 44–6, 88
   Chronic, 38
   Complementary therapies, 70
   Conventional treatment, 53, 55, 58
   Counselling, 98
   Environment, 40
   Writing, 105–6
   See also PTSD and Highly Sensitive Person
Support groups, forums and helplines 95–8

Therapy, 103, 52–64
   acupuncture, 71
   behavioural activation, 67

cognitive analytical, 59
cognitive behavioural, 54–5, 60, 62, 64–5, 67, 97
complimentary, 69–74
ego-orientated individual, 58
family, 56–7
focal psychodynamic, 53–4
group, 61, 95–7
humanistic, 59
hydrotherapy, 24, 72–3
massage and aromatherapy, 71
nutritional, 60, 79
psychoanalysis, 55–6
psychodynamic, 56
psychotherapy, 53, 55, 56, 58, 62, 119–20
writing as, 105–7